Taking Part

The Consumer's Guide to the Hospital

Taking Part

The Consumer's Guide to the Hospital

DONALD M. VICKERY, M.D.

THE CENTER FOR CORPORATE HEALTH, INC.
Oakton, Virginia 22124

Cover design by Julie Young, ProType, Great Falls, Virginia

Printed in the United States of America
Library of Congress Catalog Card Number: 86-70387

ISBN 0-9616506-0-5

89 10 9 8 7 6 5 4

"No one is as interested in your illness as you are."

William Nolen, M.D.,
author of *The Making of a Surgeon*

Acknowledgements

These brief acknowledgements are inadequate rewards for the generous contributions made toward the creation of the book. The efforts of each of the contributors named below is all the more remarkable since each has an impossibly full schedule. I really don't know how they found time for yet another task, but I am most grateful that they did.

Those who reviewed the manuscript far exceeded my expectations in the richness of their comments. Not only did they detect errors and omissions, they provided invaluable insights and suggestions. Their reviews have already laid the groundwork for an expanded program to assist individuals in making decisions about hospitalization and surgery. Thus, I owe a special debt to those who undertook the difficult task of reviewing a very rough draft: Robert W. Bradshaw; Grace H. Chickadonz, R.N., Ph.D.; J. Jarrett Clinton, M.D.; Richard L. Doyle, M.D.; James F. Fries, M.D.; Willis B. Goldbeck; Gilbert L. Gordon, M.D.; Larry A. Green, M.D.; Edith P. Gunnels; G. Timothy Johnson, M.D., M.P.H.; Kathryn Kelly; Michael J. Manley; Eugene G. McCarthy, M.D., M.P.H.; Robert M. Neiswanger; Kenneth R. Pelletier, Ph.D.; John C. Robinson, M.D.; George Sheehan, M.D.; and C. Craig Wright, M.D.

Special gratitude goes to those who labored so hard to turn my scribblings into something intelligible, and who have made numerous independent contributions in both research and writing. Janis Oppelt and Catherine Reef have demonstrated a formidable combination of talents in writing, editing, researching, and book design. Joe Vitek also deserves special thanks for preparing the chapter illustrations. Lanie King has demonstrated the range of her talent by managing the book production process as publisher and actually producing the manuscript as well.

Finally, I want to thank G. Michael Lynch, M.D., for encouraging and demonstrating good doctor-patient communication.

Why This Book?

Today's hospitals are a wonderful resource. They provide emergency care and make complex surgical procedures possible.

But the key to using hospitals well is using them wisely. Every one of us will probably have to make a decision about using the hospital at some time in our lives. Although we make these decisions with advice from our doctors, we cannot participate effectively in the decision-making process without an understanding of the benefits, risks, and costs involved. We need to be aware of our alternatives.

Most people have not received this kind of information before. They tend to overestimate the benefits of using the hospital and underestimate the risks. And they certainly can't consider alternatives if they don't know they exist.

Informed consent is the basis for hospital use; it is more than a form or a legal concept. It is patients deciding on treatment on the basis of sound, complete information. The goal of this book, then, is to give you the basic information you need to take part effectively in making decisions about the hospital.

Whose side are we on?

Yours!

If this book was provided to you by your employer, it is natural to wonder if it is meant mostly to save your company money.

Not so. Our concern is with your health. It is the plain truth that if you are healthy and use the hospital wisely, you are the main beneficiary.

Using the hospital wisely means not using it when you don't need to and, just as important, being sure to use it when it is appropriate. In fact, there will be times when we advocate spending more on medical care, such as when we recommend getting a second opinion.

But if the mention of cost still troubles you, simply ignore it. The choices suggested here are determined by the health benefits and risks to you. Saving money is just an extra benefit of making good decisions.

Can we be on your side without being against hospitals and doctors? Of course! You should use hospitals when you need to. They just are *not* good for *everything* that ails you.

How should people use this book?

Not by reading it from cover to cover.

Some of the information in this book is *general,* pertaining to such broad topics as when the hospital should be used, how to select a doctor or hospital, and the rights and responsibilities of patients. The general sections provide a good background for everyone. Since we can't know for certain when we will be faced with a decision about using the hospital, it makes sense to be informed.

Other sections are *specific,* giving information about hospitalization and treatment options for particular illnesses and conditions. You can refer to these sections if you need to make a decision about a specific illness or condition and need more information.

Therefore, we recommend that you read Part I, The Decision; Part II, Ambulatory Surgery and Emergencies; and Part III, The Hospital, before you are faced with a decision. It is a good idea to be familiar with the rest of the book to make it easier to use when you need it.

Contents

Preface

There are no courses in medical school on the costs, risks, and benefits of hospitals. As a rule, medical students arrive in the hospital for their clinical training with no more information on these subjects than any other American of comparable age. I was no exception; my ignorance of the risks of hospitalization was nearly complete. My introduction to the subject was memorable, if not dramatic.

I had completed the examination of an elderly woman, the mother of a doctor, in the emergency room. I was certain that she had pneumonia; she clearly was sick, although not in a great deal of distress. In discussing the case with the supervising physician, I recommended that she be hospitalized, but noted that the patient had said, "I don't want to come in the hospital. I might die."

I expected that the supervising physician would dismiss this as an uninformed and irrational fear. To my surprise, he replied, "Well, she certainly is right about that. Let's talk with her and see what we can work out."

The patient was started on antibiotics. She returned to her home and was cared for through a combination of phone calls and visits to her doctor's office.

Later I suggested to the supervising physician that this approach was possible because the patient, being the mother of a physician, somehow had more knowledge and skills in medicine than the average person. Again I was surprised at the response. "On the contrary, I don't think her son has tried to teach her much medicine. But he did tell her to avoid the hospital if she can. A patient without that kind of advice may have insisted upon being admitted to the hospital. And, if the patient insisted, I suspect that we would have done it."

This episode introduced me to two important concepts not taught in class: (1) Good physicians believe that even the best hospitals have risks that are to be avoided if possible, and (2) what the patient wants is important in determining whether someone is hospitalized or not. Another episode illustrated another truth not taught in medical school.

I have been fortunate enough never to have been hospitalized. My wife has done her best to make up for this gap in my experience. She has had five major surgical procedures; and indeed, without good surgeons and good hospitals, she would not be alive today. During one of these hospitalizations, a nurse brought my wife's roommate a collection of pills that were obviously different from the medication she had been taking. Nevertheless, the roommate was about to take the pills, saying, "My doctor knows best."

My wife strongly suggested that the orders should be checked, and the nurse agreed. As the nurse left the room to check the medication orders, the roommate said to my wife, "You know, if I don't take these pills, both the doctor and the nurse will be mad."

She promptly swallowed the pills. As it turned out, a mistake had been made. The wrong pills had been given to the patient, and they contained very powerful drugs. Fortunately, she suffered no long-lasting problems from having taken the medication. But the lessons were clear: (1) Mistakes do happen, and (2) patients are anxious to please doctors and nurses, even to the point of not using common sense.

There are other episodes too painful to recall in detail: The bouncy seven-year-old who came to have his tonsils out but never left the hospital alive; the physician who sought to avoid a stroke by having surgery, but suffered a massive stroke during the surgery and died without recovering consciousness.

I have seen the hospital from both sides. It is neither all good nor all bad. It saves lives and it takes them. It has the capacity for great good, but it can do harm as well. We should respect the hospital for its power. We owe it to ourselves to understand how best to use that power for our own benefit.

This book is about using the hospital for your greatest benefit. If this is to be accomplished, you must *take part* in decisions about hospitalization and surgery, and *take part* in your own care. The noted surgeon, author *and* patient, Dr. William Nolen, has put it simply yet eloquently: "No one is as interested in your illness as you are."

Doctors, nurses, and other health professionals must divide their attention among many patients. You have the advantage of being able to concentrate on the care of just one patient. Use the power of your undivided attention to make your medical care the best there is.

D.M.V.
Reston, Virginia
April 1986

Part I

THE DECISION

"Where do I begin?"

Unfortunately, there is no magic formula for making the often complex decisions about hospitalization that many people face. The more information we have, the more likely we are to make a good decision. But sometimes it's hard to know where to start.

Part I of this book is designed to give you the basics. It helps you recognize those situations in which hospitalization is appropriate and those in which it is not; it lets you know that there are hazards to hospitalization and tells you what they are; it outlines your rights and responsibilities as a patient (maybe you didn't know you had any); and it lets you know that you are not alone—there are any number of individuals, organizations, and other resources to help you make decisions and provide support.

You are entirely capable of making good decisions about the hospital. So have confidence in yourself, and get a good understanding of the basics.

1

To Go Or Not To Go

None of us takes the prospect of being hospitalized lightly. Unfortunately, this is not the same as saying that we are well prepared when the question of hospitalization arises or that we participate effectively in this important decision. Too often, hospitals are used unnecessarily, causing needless risks and expense. The best and safest use of hospitals requires the active participation of an informed patient.

How the Doctor Sees the Decision to Put You in the Hospital

The doctor's reasons for admitting individuals to the hospital can be divided into three categories:

- Specific
- Nonspecific
- Social.

Specific Indications for Hospitalization

These indications can also be divided into three categories:

1. **Complex surgical or medical therapy.** We readily understand that the hospital is the place for operations such as open-heart surgery. It is also true that some non-

surgical therapies require the special resources of the hospital.

2. **Monitoring.** The hospital may be used to observe the patient closely in order to gather information on the illness and to be ready to provide therapy if needed. The coronary care unit's role in monitoring persons who might have heart disease is the most visible example of this type of hospitalization.

3. **Diagnosis.** Certain diagnostic tests (usually complex X-ray procedures) may require hospitalization.

Great changes are occurring in all three of these areas. The latest information suggests that sometimes the therapy, monitoring, or diagnostic test is not needed at all. More commonly, there are new alternatives to the suggested procedure.

Perhaps most importantly, there is an increasing acceptance of performing many surgical and medical procedures outside the hospital. *Ambulatory* (walk in, walk out) surgery has increased markedly in recent years, as has the capacity for monitoring patients and performing diagnostic tests outside the hospital. Here are some examples:

- Many surgeons routinely perform hernia operations on an ambulatory basis. (See Chapter 10.)
- A small device called a Holter monitor can make, on magnetic tape, a continuous recording of the heartbeat (electrocardiogram) for 24 hours or more. The patient can wear the Holter monitor as he or she goes about normal activities at home or work.
- New equipment and improved procedures make almost any diagnostic test or X-ray possible on an ambulatory basis. In fact, when these tests are done in the hospital, it is usually because the patient must be hospitalized for other reasons.

It used to be that tests were covered by the patient's insurance only if they were performed in the hospital. Fortunately, most medical insurance now covers outpatient diagnostic testing in order to remove the incentive of using the hospital for testing only. This removes the temptation to risk our health, by being hospitalized, just to save money.

Nonspecific Indications for Hospitalization

Nonspecific reasons for hospitalization are often related to what might be called the "uncertainty principle." Faced with an acute and potentially serious illness, the physician may decide upon hospitalization if there is uncertainty as to the nature and course of the illness. The intention here is straightforward—to "play it safe" by admitting the patient to the hospital. The patient may be monitored and therapy may be administered, if necessary, while diagnostic tests for bringing the illness under control are performed. As discussed below, the difficulty here is knowing whether hospitalization is really the safest and best option.

Social Indications for Hospitalization

Social reasons frequently play a real and important role in the decision to hospitalize. Since these reasons are not a part of the medical reasoning involved in admission, it is often difficult to obtain precise information on them. Most often, the situation is one in which the illness does not require the level of care offered by the hospital, but the patient has no place to go for the level of care that *is* needed. A common example is the elderly patient with a flare-up of a chronic disease who needs some care, but who lives alone and has no family or friends to provide the care. Sadly, social reasons may also include abusive home situations in which a person is hospitalized simply as a way of escaping harm.

How Patients See the Decision to Enter the Hospital

Patients have a different perspective on the reasons for their admission. Their perspective and their attitudes are reflected in the way they describe the reason for admission. When a specific indication is present, patients will often say, "My doctor said I needed an operation," or, "They were doing tests on me." The nonspecific reason often reflects its connection with uncertainty—"I was really sick, and they didn't know what was wrong." A social reason may come through with disarming simplicity—"I needed someone to take care of me." Often the patient sees hospitalization as something decided upon by others and for which there were no alternatives.

Occasionally, a patient may claim to have been hospitalized because, "I needed a rest." A comment such as this is worrisome and upsetting to all of us who are concerned with the appropriate use of hospitals. As we shall see, the hospital is no place to get a rest, and the attempt to use it for this purpose is both wrong and dangerous.

Deciding to Use the Hospital

We will concentrate on your role, as the patient, in the decision to use the hospital. Hoping that someone else will take over your responsibility is unreasonable and risky. While it is traditional to emphasize the doctor's decisions with regard to the hospital, the truth is that you play a critical role in these decisions.

Patient Participation and Responsibility

From the viewpoints of both the law and medical ethics, it is the patient who agrees to be hospitalized, to have surgery, to take a drug, to undergo a diagnostic test, etc. This means that *you* are the ultimate decision maker. But regardless of the legal or ethical implications, if you are to have the best chance of using the hospital appropriately and safely, you must participate effectively in the decisions that are made.

This is not to say that physicians, nurses, and hospital personnel do not have responsibilities. They are obligated to be competent and skillful in the services that they offer, to provide you with the information you need to make *your* decision, and to be prudent in making technical decisions beyond your competence. This is as it should be. But remember, *you* are agreeing to the hospitalization and to whatever therapies, tests, or procedures are used. The only exceptions arise when decisions must be made and it is unreasonable or impossible to obtain your consent; a classic example of such a situation is emergency care rendered to an unconscious patient.

Patient Attitudes

Many of us feel more comfortable with a passive approach to the decision to enter the hospital. We conceive of ourselves as simply responding to "doctor's orders." By putting ourselves in the hands of a good physician, we escape responsibility and avoid disturbing information about our medical problem or the risks of hospitalization. It is comforting to believe that if we have a good doctor and do what we are told, everything will work out fine. It is also unrealistic. Even if you have the best doctor in the world, there still is a significant risk of disability and even death. Believing that you needn't be actively involved in your own medical care can only increase the risks.

Costs, Risks, and Benefits of Hospitalization

Every time someone is admitted to the hospital, a decision has been made that the benefits or potential benefits outweigh the costs and risks. It may come as a surprise, then, that the costs, risks, and benefits of different types of medical care, including hospitalization, have not received a great deal of study.

Here are some things we do know about the risks of hospitalization:

- Dr. Leighton Cluff and his associates at Johns Hopkins Hospital found that 97 out of 714 patients (13.6 percent) admitted to the medical service suffered a problem due to medication after admission. Six of these patients died as a result of this.

- A British survey found that 18 percent of the persons admitted to a general medical hospital suffered some undesirable consequence of drug therapy. These adverse drug reactions caused 25 percent of the deaths that occurred during the study.
- An extensive study at Yale University found that the death rate associated with hospitalization was 1.6 percent and that 20 percent of the patients studied suffered some sort of mishap or disability during the stay. These figures were obtained after excluding the problems due to errors by hospital staff. In other words, these figures are an approximation of the **inherent risks of hospitalization when everything is done right.**

These striking figures suggest that admission to the hospital is associated with a death rate of about 1 percent. To be sure, your odds are affected by your general level of health and your specific problems. But still, these are figures that command respect and underscore the need for caution where the hospital is concerned.

The benefits of hospitalization depend on the reasons for hospitalization, of course. Hospitals do save lives. Coronary care units (CCUs), for example, are estimated to reduce deaths due to heart attack (myocardial infarction) by about 5 percent overall. But there are important exceptions even when hospitalization is the best general rule. To use the CCU example, it appears that elderly persons with uncomplicated heart attacks actually do better at home than in the CCU.

Hospital costs are simply unbelievable. Average costs of more than $400 per day are the rule. Hospital bills in excess of $10,000 for a stay of a few days are not uncommon. In 1984, it is estimated that we spent $165.7 billion on hospitals.

This is almost half of everything spent on medical care. Hospital costs account for 70 percent to 80 percent of your medical insurance premium. Regardless of how you and your employer divide that premium, *you pay*. Money used by the employer for medical insurance can't be used for wages or other benefits.

Finally, almost no one who has been in a hospital thinks of it as very restful. For those who may wonder why, we offer this:

A nurse admitted to a hospital as a patient kept track of the persons entering her "semi-private" room. She counted an average of 56 such interruptions per 24 hours—and at all hours of the day and night!

The old joke about being awakened to be given a sleeping pill is no joke.

A Word About Admissions

In discussing a possible hospitalization, don't be too shocked if your physician suggests that you be admitted as an emergency patient. Your doctor may do this to avoid a delay in getting you a bed. To hospitals, there are only two major types of admissions: elective and emergency (sometimes referred to as urgent). In fact, most admissions to a medical service are urgent admissions since they are not planned in advance as elective surgery can be. Perhaps elective and nonelective admission would be better terms to use.

The recommendation of an emergency admission almost never means that there is no time for questions. You should still find out about benefits, risks, and alternatives. Usually there is time for a second opinion although these are much less common than in elective surgery. In short, don't let the word "emergency" scare you. Be an active partner in the management of your care.

When to Go In and When to Come Home

It used to be that patients requiring surgery were routinely admitted to the hospital the day before surgery was scheduled so that all the necessary testing could be done and patients could consult with anaesthesiologists and any other specialists who might be participating in their care.

While this arrangement sounds convenient, it has its drawbacks. For one thing, it assumes that the tests will not uncover anything the doctors don't already know; if they do, surgery is likely to be postponed and the patient will end up spending several days in the hospital unnecessarily. For another, even an extra night in the hospital means exposure to the inherent risks of hospitalization (see Chapter 2).

A newer approach is to do all testing and consulting outside the hospital in the days prior to surgery. The patient can then arrive at the hospital on the morning surgery is scheduled, having spent the night more comfortably at home. Patients must remember not to have anything to eat or drink after midnight, to assure that the stomach is empty.

Each chapter in this book that discusses a specific reason for hospitalization has a section on costs. These sections will tell you the *optimal* length of stay for that procedure or condition and the *average* length of stay. The optimal length of stay means the ideal—how long you need to stay if everything goes well. The average length of stay includes patients who stay longer, sometimes because of complications.

Sometimes people are kept in the hospital when they really could be at home. For example, people who have had surgery and are able to tolerate a liquid diet don't need to stay in the hospital until they have progressed to solid food. Once the digestive system is back in action, the progression to solid food is assured. Patients can also go home with catheters and other postsurgical aids if they so desire. If you are willing to take more responsibility for your postoperative care earlier than your doctor originally recommended, ask about this.

Your medical insurance may even help pay for home health care.

Finally, you don't have to be discharged in the morning. If your doctor doesn't discharge you during morning rounds, it doesn't mean you have to wait around until the next day. If you are feeling up to going home at any time during the day, speak up. The staff may very well confirm your opinion, and you can be on your way.

The Survivor's Rules for Deciding on Hospitalization

Rule #1: Ask the right questions.

To be an effective participant in the hospitalization decision, there are three questions that you must ask about the reasons for entering the hospital.

1. Are the therapies, monitoring, or diagnostic procedures necessary?
2. Are there alternatives to the therapies, monitoring, or diagnostic procedures that can be used?
3. Can the therapies, monitoring, or diagnostic tests be performed without hospitalization?

Often the answers to these questions make it clear that you have some options. Frequently, one of these options is to do nothing now but wait and see. In any event, the next step is to determine the cost, risk, and benefit of each of the options to the greatest extent possible. In our experience, patients have been most surprised to learn first that they have options, and second that the costs, risks, and benefits of the options are not precisely known. While medical science may not be able to answer all your questions, the more you know about your options, the better your chances are for a long and healthy life.

Rule #2: Accept some uncertainty, but ask the questions anyway.

If we know less than we would like about the specific indications for hospitalization, we are even more hard pressed for data with respect to the nonspecific reasons for hospitalization. If there is uncertainty as to the nature of the problem, there must also be uncertainty as to the benefits and risks of hospitalization. Circumstances vary a great deal from patient to patient. Nevertheless, the central question remains: Do the potential benefits outweigh the risks? Again, you may be surprised to find that there are options, and that the available information does not allow one to know exactly what is the best course of action.

Rule #3: Social indications for hospitalization require social solutions.

In almost all instances, if the care needed can be obtained outside the hospital, it is safer and less expensive to do so. It unnecessarily risks the life and health of the patient to use the hospital for a reason other than the need for services that only a hospital can provide.

Rule #4: Never, ever, seek to be hospitalized to get a rest.

2

Infection, Inactivity, Inherent Risks, and Incorrect Actions—The Hidden Hazards of Hospitalization

It is often said that doctors are the worst patients. Maybe yes and maybe no, but they are smart about one thing—they avoid the hospital unless there is no other choice. They know that the hospital is a hazardous environment. Working there has its risks, but it is nothing like being a patient.

The hazards that the doctor fears may be hidden to the average patient. If it's time for you to consider hospitalization, it's time to open up your eyes to the *terrible Is*.

Infection

One of the earliest and most important studies of infectious disease concluded that hospitalization distinctly increased the risk of infection. The Hungarian obstetrician Ignaz Semmelweis noted more than 100 years ago that many more mothers died during childbirth when the delivery occurred in the hospital than when it occurred in the home. These deaths were due to childbed fever (puerperal sepsis). He later demonstrated that the risks could be reduced by simply having doctors and nurses wash their hands before and after deliveries.

But the risk could not be eliminated by those measures then, and it hasn't been eliminated today by the use of antibiotics and other modern medical practices. Hospital infections continue to be a major problem for the following reasons:

1. There are a lot of "bugs" in the hospital. As patients, visitors, and staff come into the hospital, they bring their own complement of bacteria and viruses. And, of course, some of the patients are admitted because they already have an infection. The simple fact is that you have a greater chance of encountering a new "bug" in the hospital than in almost any other situation.

2. The widespread use of antibiotics in the hospital causes some of the "bugs" to become particularly nasty. The infections caused by bacteria that have developed resistance to antibiotics are very difficult to treat.

3. Hospital routines provide opportunity for infection. You will be cared for by a staff that is also caring for other patients, which means that the spread of infectious organisms is a constant possibility. Further, routine procedures such as injections or intravenous therapy may involve breaching the body's first line of defense against infection, the skin.

4. In 1985, a study of hospital infections concluded that they are a major threat and that the biggest problem was *still* getting doctors and nurses to wash their hands!

Hospital staffs are aware of all these risks, of course, and are required to use procedures to minimize them. But the risks cannot be eliminated, and some hospitals do a better job of minimizing them than others.

Inactivity

One of the most harmful myths of our times is that rest is always good for what ails you. We now know that putting someone to bed as a form of treatment is to be avoided if at all possible. The simple truth is that **the body requires activity to remain healthy.** Hospital routines make adequate activity difficult even if you have not been told to stay in bed.

Inactivity creates a number of problems:

1. It increases the risk of infection, especially infections of the lungs.
2. It decreases your conditioning, making you less able to deal with the stress of hospitalization and any procedures that you may undergo.
3. It contributes to depression and malaise—real hazards of hospitalization.

Most importantly, a healthy circulatory system requires exercise and activity. Inactivity increases the risk of inflammation within veins (thrombophlebitis), especially in the legs. Thrombophlebitis may cause swelling and considerable pain, but its greatest hazard lies in the formation of blood clots that can break free and be carried by the circulating blood to the lungs (pulmonary emboli). We now know that pulmonary emboli are fairly common. Small ones may cause few symptoms and are rarely diagnosed. But if the clots are large or there are many of them, they may seriously impede the flow of blood to the lungs and cause severe problems, including death.

Sudden death from pulmonary embolism seems much more tragic when it occurs during an unnecessary hospitalization, as in the case of a young man who died while undergoing traction therapy for low back pain. Bed rest may be necessitated by pain in the beginning, but three weeks of bed rest (as in this case) is clearly excessive. The risks to this young man could have been reduced, although not eliminated, had a different approach been taken to treat his back pain.

You will have to work at being active in the hospital.

1. Walk, walk, walk!
2. Do whatever else (bending, pushups, etc.) that your condition permits.

It is essential to stay as active as possible within any limits imposed by your medical problem. It can save your life.

One final note: Special elastic stockings are sometimes used to try to decrease the risk of thrombophlebitis and, therefore, the risk of pulmonary embolism. They are controversial and, if used improperly, actually may increase the risk of thrombophlebitis. Do not put your faith in these stockings. They are no substitute for exercise and activity.

Inherent Risks

All of medicine's tools carry built-in risks. These risks are not due to inappropriate use or errors by the hospital staff. Hospitalization means that more of these tools will be used, and the risks to you increase accordingly.

Drugs

Drugs constitute a major portion of the risk in hospitalization. Consider the following:

- Dr. Leighton Cluff and his associates at Johns Hopkins Hospital followed 714 patients admitted to general medical beds. They found that 122 patients (17 percent) suffered 184 adverse drug reactions. Drug reactions were responsible for 5 percent of these admissions in the first place. Six patients died as a result of hospital-acquired drug reactions.
- In a second study, the same group found that certain drugs were more likely to be associated with adverse reactions. Barbiturates, codeine, penicillins, and thiazide diuretics produced 70 percent of the drug problems despite the fact that

they accounted for only 17 percent of all the medications that had been administered.

- A British survey found that 193 out of 731 patients (18 percent) admitted to a general medical hospital suffered undesirable consequences of drug therapy. Seventeen of the 67 deaths that occurred among these patients were due to adverse drug reactions.
- Most drug reactions are related directly to the chemical effect of the drug and only a small percentage (less than 10 percent) is due to drug allergies.

The bottom line is simple: Every drug carries a risk. Avoid drugs unless you are convinced that the benefits outweigh the risks.

X-rays

Exposure to radiation increases the risk of cancer. The amount of radiation you receive during X-ray procedures depends on the type of procedure and whether or not adequate protective shielding (lead aprons, etc.) is used. The amount of radiation you receive will vary from a relatively small amount in examinations such as a plain chest X-ray to a large amount in procedures that involve taking many X-rays or the use of *fluoroscopy,* a technique in which a continuous exposure to X-rays is necessary so that the image may be viewed on a television screen.

While the effects of X-rays due to radiation exposure become apparent over the long term, a more immediate threat comes from substances injected or ingested in order to make certain body structures visible on the X-ray. These chemicals, referred to as *contrast agents or "dyes,"* can cause serious allergic reactions that in many ways resemble the reactions some people suffer after bee stings. These reactions may cause relatively minor problems, such as hives, but they can cause circulatory collapse and death.

Laboratory Tests

The risks in laboratory tests are much more hidden than those involved with drugs or X-rays. After all, it may hurt a little to have the blood taken or be inconvenient to collect the urine sample, but it seems that these do little harm.

The problem with laboratory tests is that they may give a false positive or a false negative reading. This could result in your being misdiagnosed and subjected to unnecessary therapies or procedures, or in your being denied appropriate treatments or procedures. **The risk of false results is highest when there is no real indication for the test, i.e., when tests are done as a part of "routine" admission or presurgery testing.**

Incorrect Actions

The people who work in hospitals use powerful tools—tools that can hurt as well as help. And sometimes people make mistakes.

You have heard the horror stories—the wrong patient operated on, the wrong leg amputated, the good eye removed, the wrong drug injected. In many of these cases, there is reason to believe that negligence may have been involved. But negligence is not required. There are such things as honest mistakes, and the best doctors, the best nurses, and the best hospital staffs can make them.

For your own protection, accept the notion of an honest mistake. Your best defense against the honest mistake is to be alert; to understand what is happening to you; to ask questions; to make sure that the drug, the X-ray, or the procedure is indicated and one that is intended for you. This is also your best defense against negligence, but you do not have to suspect incompetence to protect yourself. You do not have to be paranoid to believe that people can make mistakes that will hurt you. You just have to be smart. Remember, you are the person most concerned with your health and well-being.

Reducing Your Risks

There are three essentials for reducing the threat of inherent risks:

1. **Make sure that there is a valid indication for every test, X-ray, or drug.** Do not accept any of these because they are "routine." Studies have shown that such laboratory tests and X-rays do not produce any benefit and do pose a threat to you. Do not accept a routine pain or sleeping medication unless *you* feel that the benefit outweighs the risk.

2. **Insist that proper shielding be used during any X-ray procedure.** It is especially important that reproductive organs (ovaries, testes) be shielded. Remember that X-rays can only look at one portion of the body at a time and that usually this is a small portion. The rest of the body should be protected.

3. **Know about your case.** This is your life. Be sure that you know what is being done and why. Ask questions and remember that *you* must give consent to your treatment.

3
Patients' Rights and Responsibilities

"Doctor's Orders." Most of us are comfortable with this term despite the fact that we don't like to be ordered around. This is due in part to the fact that our culture, like many others, has given physicians a unique authority in their relationships with patients. Perhaps more importantly, it reflects our desire to put ourselves in the hands of a wise and all-knowing physician who relieves us of responsibility and reassures us that everything will be all right. This may be a comforting thought, but it is a myth. Believing in this myth can have very uncomfortable results.

Informed consent is a far newer concept that reflects an essential truth about your dealings with health professionals in the hospital. Patients are entitled to accept or reject health care on the basis of their own personal values and in the pursuit of their own personal goals. Anything that is done to or for you in the hospital is done on the basis that you have agreed to it and that you understood what you were doing when you gave your consent.

Unfortunately, the practice of informed consent may be far removed from the theory. Both patients and health professionals may put too much emphasis on forms and getting signatures on them.

An informed consent statement should be regarded as a tool to foster understanding between patients and professionals. It is not a contract and your signature does not mean that you have relinquished your rights and responsibilities with respect to your care. Sadly, many informed consent statements serve only to confuse and intimidate. Such forms neither serve their primary purpose nor protect the hospital or health professionals in any way. Indeed, it is the responsibility of health professionals to inform and share decision making with the patient. Unclear or complex informed consent statements actually increase the liability of hospitals or professionals. Under no circumstances does a signature absolve the hospital or its staff of their responsibilities.

It is also true that both patients and physicians appear not to appreciate the full meaning of informed consent. A survey by the President's Commission for the Study of Ethical Problems in Medicine found that the public was confused about the meaning of informed consent. While 44 percent of those surveyed said informed consent meant the patient was informed, only 10 percent mentioned that the risks should be specified. Less than 1 percent mentioned that alternatives would be presented. Some people expressed very little understanding at all of informed consent, identifying it simply as a form or as giving consent to termination of treatment.

The physicians surveyed did only a little better. Fifty-nine percent said it meant informing the patient about condition and treatment; 47 percent mentioned disclosing treatment risks to the patient. Only 26 percent mentioned the patient giving permission, and only 9 percent indicated that the patient could make a choice or state a preference about treatment.

While these results are disappointing, they are understandable. Informed consent is a phrase that reflects the concept of shared decision making—a process that can be complex and that requires effort from both the patient and the health professional. It is also a process that offers many opportunities for misunderstanding. Despite its difficulties, shared decision making is an absolute necessity. It is the only way the patient's right to accept or reject health care can be merged with the health professional's expertise and responsibilities. There is no easy formula for sharing decision making or for guidelines that work in every situation. Understanding your rights and responsibilities is the best guide to shared decision making.

PATIENTS' RIGHTS ARE BASED ON THE PRINCIPLE THAT PATIENTS MAY ACCEPT OR REJECT HEALTH CARE ON THE BASIS OF THEIR OWN PERSONAL VALUES AND IN FURTHERANCE OF THEIR OWN PERSONAL GOALS, AND TO DO THIS EFFECTIVELY THEY REQUIRE UNDERSTANDABLE INFORMATION. THESE RIGHTS INCLUDE:

1. **The right to be informed as to the problem, alternative approaches to the problem, and the expected risks and benefits of each approach.**
2. **The right to make choices when appropriate.**
3. **The right to have health professionals assume their responsibility for integrating shared decision making into health care.**

PATIENTS' RESPONSIBILITIES ARE BASED ON THE PRINCIPLE THAT INFORMED AND INTELLIGENT PARTICIPATION IN THE DECISION-MAKING PROCESS IS REQUIRED. THESE RESPONSIBILITIES INCLUDE:-

1. **The patient must understand that the information presented may include uncertainties and/or unpleasant realities.**
2. **A patient competent to make decisions shall not assign this responsibility to family members, friends, doctors, nurses, or others.**

3. The patient cannot demand services that violate the bounds of acceptable practice or would draw upon a limited resource for which the patient has no claim. The patient must not demand that a particular health professional provide a service that would violate that professional's own deeply held moral beliefs.

4

Resources—Where to Go for Help

No one needs to face hospitalization alone. People frequently feel overwhelmed or cut off from those around them when faced with a serious health problem. Actually, it is not as difficult as it may at first seem to get the information and support you need to make good decisions about surgery and the hospital.

This book is an excellent resource to begin with, and a librarian can help you find others. Your doctor will provide important medical information and recommendations, as will the doctor you consult for a second opinion. Your family and friends are a frequently underestimated network for support both during and after your hospital stay. Finally, a number of volunteer organizations, government agencies, and nonprofit groups provide information and support.

Doctors

When talking with your doctor about your medical condition, it is important not to be shy. If you don't understand something he or she tells you, ask to have it explained more clearly. Be sure that your doctor makes clear the benefits, risks, and costs of hospitalization and/or surgery, and that he or she discusses all treatment options with you.

Getting a second opinion is often a good idea when hospitalization is recommended, particularly if surgery is proposed. Second opinions have become common practice, and getting one is something your doctor expects you to do. Therefore, don't feel uncomfortable about saying that you plan to do this. Your doctor will be able to pass along test results and other information to the doctor providing the second opinion and will be available for consultation about your condition if necessary. Remember that your doctor probably provides second opinions for other doctors' patients.

A second doctor may consider certain aspects of your case quite differently or point out something your doctor has overlooked. Getting a second opinion is one time when it is good to spend more money on medical care. If you decide not to have surgery because of a second opinion, you have saved yourself discomfort and risk in addition to money. However, if the second doctor confirms your doctor's opinion, you have the security of knowing you have made a sensible decision in opting for surgery or hospitalization.

The People Around You

Many times, family members and friends feel a need to do something actively to help you get well. Don't be afraid to ask them to take part in planning for your care and recovery.

While you are in the hospital, family members can keep you company and contribute to your comfort by doing such simple things as adjusting your bed, calling a nurse for you, or bringing you a snack from the cafeteria. They can help the nursing staff understand your needs and preferences, and they can take part in your care if they are willing.

Helpful relatives and friends can aid in your recovery at home by preparing meals, helping you out of bed, and providing other needed assistance. Having this kind of help at home may make it possible for you to leave the hospital sooner and recover in familiar, comfortable surroundings.

The one caution in asking friends and family for help is to be realistic in what you expect of them. Be sure that no one person bears too much of the responsibility for your care.

Organizations

All kinds of organizations exist to provide information and support to people with medical problems. These range from large national organizations such as The American Cancer Society and The American Diabetes Association to local support groups for people who have undergone specific types of surgery.

Many people don't realize that large national organizations frequently have chapters located throughout the country. In this way they can provide needed services to people who don't live near their national headquarters.

Your doctor or someone on the hospital staff may be able to tell you how to get in touch with an organization that can be of help to you. You can also call your city, county, or state public health department for the names, addresses, and phone numbers of organizations in your area. Your local medical society is another possible source for this information.

Part II

AMBULATORY SURGERY AND EMERGENCIES

People requiring ambulatory surgery or the services of the emergency room are not actually admitted to the hospital, but they do have important decisions to make.

Many procedures that once required admission to the hospital are now being done on an ambulatory, or outpatient, basis. Hernia operations are a good example. Sometimes people are confused about what ambulatory surgery means and when it is appropriate.

Emergency rooms provide quick, essential care to seriously ill or injured people. Frequently they save lives. Most people who use emergency rooms are capable of participating in the decision-making process even though they may not be admitted to the hospital. Therefore, it pays to know what to do. It also pays to know when not to use the emergency room. Unnecessary visits cost time and money.

Ambulatory surgery and emergency rooms are two health-care options that could benefit from better utilization. The first could be used more, and the second could definitely be used less. It is certainly worth your while to know how to make appropriate decisions about ambulatory surgery and the emergency room.

5

Ambulatory Surgery

Ambulatory surgery, outpatient surgery, in-and-out surgery, same-day surgery—all terms for surgery that can be done without your having to stay in the hospital. Such surgical procedures are relatively short in duration and require little or no general anaesthesia. They usually do not require opening a major body cavity (skull, chest, or abdomen), blood transfusions, or intensive postoperative care. They are unlikely to have complications that would require major surgery or hospitalization.

Physicians believe that many well known procedures (Table 5.1 on page 30) can usually be done on an ambulatory basis. There are many others (Table 5.2 on page 32) that, although they are somewhat less common, are almost always done as ambulatory surgery. Table 5.2 is intended as a reference for people contemplating surgery or another procedure so that they can determine whether this can be done on an ambulatory basis. The terms in this table are technical, but they are the terms that doctors use and that appear on medical insurance forms.

Table 5.1   Common Procedures That are Usually Performed on an Ambulatory Basis

MEDICAL TERM	DEFINITION
Adenoidectomy	Removal of the adenoids
Angiogram (including cardiac catheterization)	An X-ray of the blood vessels after injection of a contrast medium (dye)
Arthrogram	An X-ray of a joint following the injection of a contrast medium, referred to as a dye
Arthroscopy	The examination of the interior of a joint using a special instrument*
Biopsy	The removal of tissue for diagnostic examination (frequent biopsies: bone marrow, breast, nerve, prostate, lymph node, muscle, rib, liver)
Blepharoplasty	Any operation performed to correct a defect in the eyelid
Bronchoscopy	Inspection of the interior of the air passages in the lung (trachea and bronchi)*
Bunionectomy (including bilateral and hammertoe repair)	The removal of a bunion, a painful, inflamed swelling at the joint of the big toe
Carpal tunnel release or tarsal tunnel release	Surgery to relieve pressure on nerves in the wrist (carpal tunnel) or ankle (tarsal tunnel)
Cataract extraction (including implant or phacoemulsification)	Surgical removal of the lens of the eye
Colonoscopy	Visual examination of the inner surface of the colon*
Cystoscopy	Inspection of the interior of the urinary bladder and ureter*
Dilatation and curettage (D&C)	Dilation of the cervix and scraping of the endometrium (mucous membrane comprising the inner layer of the uterine wall)

Table 5.1   *(Continued)*

MEDICAL TERM	DEFINITION
Esophagogastroduoden-oscopy	Looking into the esophagus, stomach and duodenum using a special flexible tube*
Fistulectomy, anal	Removal of an abnormal passage leading from the skin to the inside of the rectum
Hemorrhoidectomy	Surgical removal of hemorrhoids
Herniorrhaphy	Surgery to repair a hernia
Hydrocelectomy	Removal of a sac of watery fluid
Laparoscopy (including tubal ligation)	Examination of the contents of abdomen and/or pelvis*
Myelography	X-ray of the spinal cord after injection of a contrast medium (dye)
Myringotomy	Making an opening in the eardrum for the purpose of draining fluid
Pilonidal cyst excision	The removal of a cyst from the area of the anus
Proctosigmoidoscopy	Direct inspection of the rectum and the sigmoid colon*
Rhinoplasty	Partial or complete repair of a defect of the nose
Septoplasty	An operation to correct defects or deformities of the nasal septum
Sigmoidoscopy	Inspection of the interior of the sigmoid colon*
Tenotomy	The surgical division of a tendon for the relief of deformities caused by the shortening of a muscle
Tonsillectomy	Removal of the tonsils
Varicocelectomy	Surgical removal of a varicocele (abnormal dilation of the veins of the spermatic cord)
Varicotomy	Surgery to cure varicose veins

*Any procedure that is performed to "examine the interior" of a joint or organ is completed with the help of some variation of an instrument known as an endoscope. This endoscope goes by various names, according to the specific procedure for which it is used.

Table 5.2   Comprehensive List of Ambulatory Procedures

If your physician recommends one of these procedures, find out if it can be done on an outpatient basis. For help with these unfamiliar medical terms, ask your doctor or nurse, or use a medical dictionary at a public library.

Abscess drainage
Acromionectomy
Adenoidectomy with or without myringotomy
Alveolectomy or alveoloplasty
Amniocentesis
Anal fistulectomy, or other anal surgery
Ankle fracture, nondisplaced, single malleolar, including manipulation or reduction
Antral puncture
Antrostomy, intranasal
Apicoectomy
Arteriogram
Arteriovenous shunt creation for hemodialysis or arteriovenous shunt irrigation, replacement or revision
Arthrodesis, fingers or toes
Arthroplasty, small joints, i.e., fingers and toes
Arthrotomy, small joints
Arthrotomy with removal of loose bodies (elbows, knees or small joints)
Avulsion of nail, complete

Bartholin cyst, excision or marsupialization
Benign neoplasm of male genitalia, excision
Blepharotomy
Blood and blood derivative transfusions
Body cast, application of
Bone marrow biopsy
Branchial cleft cyst, excision
Breast, aspiration of cyst, biopsy or excision of tumor (lumpectomy)
Bursa, removal, elbow
Bursa, infected, drainage of

Capsulectomy/capsulotomy, small joints
Cardiac catheterization
Cardioversion, elective
Central venous catheter placement for hyperalimentation

Table 5.2 *(Continued)*

Cervix:
  biopsy
  cauterization
  conization
  fulguration or laser cautery
Chalazion excision
Chemical cauterization of verruca
Chondroma, excision of
Chondroplasty by arthroscopy
Circumcision
Closed reduction of nasal fracture
Colostomy revision
Condylectomy
Condyloma acuminatam treatment
Conization biopsy
Cryotherapy
Cryotherapy with biopsy and/or with D&C
Culdoscopy/Culdocentesis
Cutaneous nerve neuroma excision
Cystourethroscopy

Dacryocystostomy
Dermabrasion of skin
Destruction of nevi, actinic keratosis or senile keratosis
Digital nerve neuroma excision
Dilation of esophagus
Dilation of vagina
Discission (needling of lens)
Dislocation, congenital, hip, childhood traction treatment
Dislocation, congenital, hip, closed reduction
Dislocation, congenital, reduction in infant
Dislocation, simple, elbow or shoulder, closed reduction
Drainage of hematoma, simple
Drainage of infected bursa
Drainage of onychia or paronychia
Duputytren's contracture fasciectomy or release

Ectropion repair
Electrosurgical destruction of lesions
Endometrial biopsy
Endoscopy
Endoscopic Retrograde Cannulation of the Pancreas (ERCP)

Table 5.2 *(Continued)*

Entropion repair
Epididymectomy
Esophageal dilation
Esotropia
Excision of skin lesions, small bone cysts and other lesions
   including:
   branchial cleft cysts
   breast tumors
   chalazions
   chondromas
   condyles
   cysts
   exostoses
   fibromas
   ganglions
   heel spurs
   lipomas
   malignant skin lesions
   mandible cysts
   melanoma without node dissection
   neuromas including Morton's and cutaneous nerve neuromas
   osteochondromas
   pilonidal cysts and sinuses
   polyps
   sebaceous cysts
   supernumerary ossicles
   turbinates
Excision of foreign body, uncomplicated
Excision of ingrown toenails
Excision of nails, partial or complete
Exostosectomy, simple, small bones
Extractions, dental, simple or multiple
Eye muscle surgery

Finger amputation
Finger joint replacement
Fingernail/toenail removal
Foreign body removal, esophagus, eye or joints
Fracture, closed reductions, small joints
Fracture of humerus, shaft
Fracture of inferior turbinate

Table 5.2 *(Continued)*

Fracture of nose
Fracture of wrist
Frenectomy
Fusion of small joints
Ganglion excision
Gingivectomy or gingivoplasty

Hallux valgus exostosectomy
Hammertoe repair w/bone resection, and tenotomies
Hand tendon repair
Hematoma, drainage
Hip joint manipulation for congenital dislocation
Humerus, shaft, fracture
Hymenectomy or hymenotomy
Hysterosalpingogram
Hysteroscopy

Incision and drainage of infection and sebaceous cysts,
    carbuncles, furuncles and other cutaneous and subcutaneous
    abscesses, including perirectal abscesses
Inguinal herniorrhaphy
Injection of peripheral nerve
Insufflation of Fallopian tubes
Intralesional injections
Intrauterine device (I.U.D.) removal
Iridectomy

Joint fusion, small joints
Joint manipulations

Keratoplasty
Keratosis, actinic or senile, destruction of

Labia, plastic revision
Laceration of tongue, repair
Lacrimal duct drainage, probing, reconstruction or splitting
Laparotomy, mini
Laryngoscopy, direct, including foreign body removal or radium
    insertion
Laryngoscopy with or without tubal ligation
Laser cautery
Leg cast, application of

Table 5.2 *(Continued)*

Lens discission
Lens extraction, external
Lens implant
Ligation of spermatic vein
Ligation or stripping of varicose veins, unilateral
Lip malignancy, excision
Lip wedge resection
Lip wound repair
Lipoma excision
Liver biopsy
Lumbar puncture
Lymph node biopsy

Malignant skin lesion, excision
Mammoplasty
Mandible cyst excision
Meatotomy
Metatarsal head excision, single
Muscle biopsy
Morton's neuroma excision

Nasal lacrimal duct probing
Nasal polypectomy
Nerve blocks, biopsies, injections, or repairs, simple
Neurectomy
Neurolysis, simple
Neuroma excision (Morton's, cutaneous or digital nerve)
Nevi, destruction of
Nose, fracture, closed reduction

Onychia, drainage of
Orchiopexy for chronic torsion
Orchidectomy
Ossicle, supernumerary, excision of
Ostectomy of fingers, toes, single metatarsal heads
Osteochondroma, excision of
Osteotomy, simple
Otoplasty
Otoscopy
Oxytocin challenge test

Paracentesis

Table 5.2 *(Continued)*

Paronychia, drainage of
Pelvic examination under anaesthesia
Perineoplasty
Perineorrhaphy
Peridontal therapy
Phalangectomy
Pilonidal sinus excision
Plantar wart, excision
Polypectomy, nasal
Polypectomy, rectal
Prostate biopsy, needle
Pterygium excision
Pulpotomy

Reduction mammoplasty
Reduction of nasal fracture, closed
Removal of impacted teeth
Renal biopsy
Repair of small lacerations including lacerations of tongue, lip or
    tendons
Revision of colostomy
Revision of enterostomy
Revision of scars
Rhytidectomy
Rib biopsy
Root canal
Rubberband hemorrhoidectomy
Ruptured extensor tendon, wrist repair

Sclerotomy for glaucoma
Sebaceous cyst, excision of
Silastic arthroplasty, toe
Sinusotomy, sinus puncture
Skin lesion excision with or without primary closure
Small skin grafts
Somatic nerve excision
Spermatocelectomy
Strabismus surgery
Syndactylism surgery
Synovectomy, simple, fingers, toes

Tarsal tunnel release

Ambulatory Surgery

Table 5.2   *(Continued)*

Tarsorrhaphy
Temporal artery biopsy or ligation
Tendon procedures including tendoplasty or tendon repair,
    tenectomy, tenotomy of hands, fingers, feet, toes or ankles,
    and tendon sheath release (DeQuervain's)
Tenosynovectomy, finger, toe, wrist, flexor or extensor tendon
    sheaths
Thoracentesis
Tissue transfer or rearrangement
Toe amputation
Toenail removal
Tongue biopsy
Tonsillectomy
Tooth extraction
Tracheostomy, elective
Transfusion, blood and blood derivative
Trigger finger tenovaginotomy
Tubal ligation
Turbinate resection
Tympanoplasty
Tympanotomy

Umbilical herniorraphy
Upper endoscopy
Urethral caruncle excision
Urethral dilatation

Vaginal biopsy, cyst or polyp excision
Vaginal dilation
Vaginal stenosis release
Vasectomy
Verruca, chemical cauterization
Vesical calculus, small cystoscopic removal
Vulvar biopsy, lesion excision, fulguration, laser cautery

Wedge resection of lip
Wrist fracture, treatment of

Zygoma reduction, simple

The advantages of ambulatory surgery are convenience, lower risk, and less cost. Most patients prefer having a specific time to have the procedure done and recuperating at home. Spending less time in the hospital means avoiding the risks associated with it, especially infection and inactivity. Finally, the costs of such surgery are, or at least should be, less than if the more expensive facilities of the hospital are used.

The increasing demand for ambulatory surgery has led to the development of ambulatory surgery centers, often referred to as surgicenters, that are completely separate from hospitals. Such facilities are designed, staffed, and organized specifically for the purpose of preparing the patient for surgery, performing the procedure safely and efficiently, and returning the patient home all in the same day.

While many hospitals have developed surgicenters, many others have set aside part of their outpatient department specifically for ambulatory surgery. If well organized, such facilities may have the advantages of the surgicenter as well as immediate access to the other facilities of the hospital if needed.

Some hospitals actually use their regular operating rooms for ambulatory surgery. However, this is usually the case only in small hospitals where no other facilities are available. Most hospital operating rooms are equipped, staffed, and organized for major surgery and are not efficient when it comes to ambulatory surgery.

Before using any ambulatory surgery facility, you should determine what arrangements for medical back-up (major surgery and/or hospitalization) have been made. The chance of a complication requiring such back-up is exceedingly small for most ambulatory surgical procedures, but it is prudent to make sure that it is available.

It is also wise to determine how your medical insurance handles ambulatory surgery. Many medical insurance plans, including Medicare and

Medicaid, have instituted procedures to insure that patients are not admitted to the hospital when the surgical procedure can be done on an ambulatory basis. Some plans also have incentives to encourage use of ambulatory surgical facilities when hospitalization is an option. Be aware that confusion sometimes arises when ambulatory surgery is performed in the hospital even if it is done in the outpatient department. It's best to determine ahead of time how the insurance plan will treat your particular case using a specific facility.

Deciding on Ambulatory Surgery

If you have the option, ambulatory surgery is your best choice because of convenience, lower risk, and less cost. Be sure that you understand what the medical back-up is and how charges for the procedure will be handled. By returning home sooner to recuperate, you will more quickly return to your normal routine.

6
Emergency Rooms

Emergency! The word itself can make you anxious. It suggests a life-and-death situation, a time to stand back and let the emergency team do whatever it has to do.

Most injuries and illnesses treated in emergency rooms do not relate to life or death. In most cases, you still must play an important role in the decisions being made.

Emergency rooms are equipped and staffed to handle life-and-death situations—major injuries, cardiac arrests, people choking on something swallowed, and so on. But about 90 percent of emergency room visits involve minor problems that are not emergencies and do not require urgent care—sore throats, minor cuts, skin rashes. This does not necessarily mean that the hospital is unhappy to see you. Indeed, most hospitals will be happy to have the income from your visit.

From your point of view, the visit to the emergency room for a minor problem may be a much less happy event. The convenience of being able to walk in may well be offset by having to wait while patients with more urgent problems receive care. The cost is substantial: You cannot set foot in most emergency rooms for less than $50, and the total bill for the emergency room, the doctor, and any tests or X-rays is likely to be in excess of $150. You will have to pay this amount directly, share the cost with your insurance, or, even if insurance covers this bill, pay for it indirectly through higher insurance rates. Most medical insurance plans have developed or are developing procedures to discourage such expensive care for minor illnesses. This usually means that you will pay all or most of the bill if you use the emergency room for a minor problem.

Making Decisions About Using the Emergency Room

It is difficult to provide strict guidelines for determining when the emergency room should be used. This is because individual situations can vary greatly and all kinds of things can happen to people. But some signs do show you that what you are faced with is a true emergency.

Major injury. The patient with a broken leg, large chest wound, or other severe injury requires immediate attention at an emergency facility.

Unconsciousness. The patient who is unconscious needs emergency care immediately.

Active bleeding. A wound that continues to bleed despite the application of pressure requires attention in order to prevent unnecessary loss of blood. Remember that vigorous bleeding can almost always be controlled by the direct application of pressure and that this is the most important part of first aid for such wounds.

Stupor or drowsiness. A practical way to determine if stupor or drowsiness requires urgent treatment is to note the patient's ability to answer questions. If the patient is not sufficiently awake to answer questions concerning what happened, then urgent action is necessary. Any child who cannot be aroused needs immediate attention.

Disorientation. Disorientation may be part of a variety of illnesses and is especially common when a high fever is present. A patient is disoriented if he or she cannot tell the date, the location, or who he or she is. Someone who has previously been alert but then becomes disoriented deserves immediate medical attention.

Shortness of breath. As a general rule, shortness of breath requires immediate attention if it occurs even when the patient is at rest. A frequent cause of shortness of breath in young people is the hyperventilation syndrome, which is not a serious concern. But if you can't be certain of the cause, seek immediate aid for shortness of breath.

Cold sweat. Cold sweat is a common effect of severe pain or illness. Sweating without other complaints is unusual; therefore, as an isolated symptom it is not likely to be serious. But a cold sweat in a patient complaining of chest pain, abdominal pain or lightheadedness indicates a need for immediate attention.

Severe pain. Severe pain is usually accompanied by other symptoms that indicate the nature of the condition; the most obvious example is pain associated with a major injury. The severity of pain depends upon the particular patient; often its magnitude is altered by emotional and psychological factors. Nevertheless, severe pain demands urgent medical attention if for no other reason than providing relief.

If a situation arises in which you are not sure of the need to make a trip to the hospital, contact your physician by telephone. He or she will question you about the patient and determine the best course to follow. Telephoning the physician is a good idea, too, if his or her office is closed and a situation develops that is not a real emergency but requires medical attention. Your doctor does not want you to suffer unnecessary discomfort and will see to it that you get the attention you need.

Part III

THE HOSPITAL

Hospitals are such powerful social institutions that it's no wonder they make people feel intimidated and helpless. Strange tests and procedures that are part of some mysterious "routine" and an endless procession of white-clad professionals cause people to wonder, "Who's in charge here?"

Part III of this book explains the roles performed by hospital personnel and provides some guidelines to follow regarding tests, medication, and other hospital "routines." These chapters are designed to give you some feeling of control in what can be an overwhelming situation.

Because many people wonder about choosing a doctor or hospital, a chapter on this subject is included. Frequently, these basic choices can determine the quality of the treatment they receive.

It should be noted that when we use the term *hospital* in this book we are talking about the general acute care hospital, the kind that is equipped to handle a variety of patients in different departments—medicine, surgery, pediatrics, etc. It is the kind of hospital that most of us are familiar with.

There are other kinds of hospitals designed to handle the needs of specific patient groups—the mentally ill and those afflicted with terminal cancer, for example. But in hospitals of all types there will be people in similar roles, and similar procedures are likely to be followed.

It is impossible to cover all situations or all kinds of hospitals in one book; however, the basic information provided here should be transferable to other types of hospitalizations.

7
The Hospital Staff

Doctors

It is very likely that you will encounter doctors other than your personal doctor when you enter the hospital. Often there is confusion about the role of other physicians. This is understandable since there are a number of different arrangements by which you may come into contact with a doctor who appears to be a part of the hospital staff.

The Medical Staff

In its most basic form, the term *medical staff* simply refers to those physicians who are permitted to practice within the hospital. It does not necessarily mean that they are employed by the hospital or even that they spend very much time there. Staffs are virtually always organized into departments by specialties (medicine, surgery, pediatrics, obstetrics and gynecology, etc.), and each of these departments has a chairman. In addition, there is usually a medical staff organization with its own officers—president, vice president, etc. Again, being chairman of the department or an officer of the medical staff does not necessarily mean that a doctor is employed by the hospital or that he or she practices primarily in the hospital.

How the staff is organized and who is on the staff are influenced mostly by the size of the hospital and whether it is a teaching hospital (one involved in training physicians through an affiliation with a medical school). A teaching hospital may be a university hospital that is owned and operated by a medical school. It may also be a community hospital that is affiliated with a medical school so that it can participate in physician training. Such an affiliation usually is undertaken because it is felt that this improves the quality of care in the hospital.

Interns and Residents

If you should be admitted to a teaching hospital, you will encounter the resident staff. These are physicians involved in post-graduate training in their chosen specialty. As such, they work in conjunction with, and under the supervision of, a senior physician who is usually referred to as the *attending physician*. Often the attending physician is also your personal physician. However, some large teaching hospitals, especially university hospitals, have two ways of organizing their medical services. The *private service* maintains the personal physician as the attending physician and uses the medical school faculty as consultants. The *teaching service* uses a medical school faculty member as the attending physician and the personal physician as a consultant.

The resident staff is just that—they reside within the hospital and are expected to provide 24-hour coverage for patients on the teaching services. You should see a great deal more of the residents than the attending physician. When you are on the teaching service, a resident assumes the role of personal physician. The role is more variable on a private service, but here, too, the resident is usually the physician in most direct contact with the patient. In any event, you should expect more direct involvement by your personal physician on a private service than on a teaching service.

You may not welcome the idea of resident physicians being involved in your care. Certainly, the involvement of additional physicians can increase the number of times you must give your medical history or be examined; teaching hospitals inevitably involve patients in more activity than nonteaching hospitals. Nevertheless, it is a nearly universally accepted proposition that teaching hospitals deliver the best medical care. You should consider this tradeoff before deciding whether or not to allow residents to be involved in your care. Also, you should know that in some teaching hospitals it is difficult or impossible to be admitted unless residents participate in your care.

Residency programs in most medical specialties run for three years. In the past, the first year was usually referred to as an internship, but this term fell out of favor in the 1960s and 1970s. Interestingly, there seems to be a developing enthusiasm for its return.

On a teaching service, you are usually assigned a first- or second-year resident as your "personal" physician. This physician works as part of a team with other first- or second-year residents who are supervised by a third-year, or senior, resident. The entire team's work is supervised by an attending physician who usually meets with the team once or twice a day and examines individual patients as necessary.

On a private service, the private attending physician makes arrangements to meet with the team concerning his or her patients once or twice a day.

Chief residents in the past were physicians who stayed for a special fourth year of residency in which they supervised the entire resident staff for a particular department (medicine, pediatrics, surgery, etc.). Today, chief residents are often third-year residents who have been selected for additional responsibility.

Hospital-Based Specialties

There are certain medical specialties that are expected to be available within the hospital. These include anaesthesia, radiology (X-rays), and pathology (blood tests, etc.). Other special services such as nuclear medicine and physical medicine may be represented as independent departments or may come under another department. While some hospitals employ physicians to provide these services, it is more common for the hospital to contract with a group of physicians for this purpose. In either instance, these physicians are likely to have their offices within the hospital, and they will provide the appropriate services should you require them. It is unlikely that you will meet the pathologist, and you may not meet the radiologist unless the X-ray procedure requires that he or she be involved. However, you certainly should meet and be examined by an anaesthesiologist if you will require anaesthesia.

Working With Your Doctors

Nearly everyone, patients and doctors alike, subscribes to the notion that there should be just one physician in charge, a quarterback for this medical team. There can be no doubt that having no one responsible for coordinating medical care would result in disaster, but the concept of just one doctor making decisions usually must take into account the necessity of involving more than one physician in your case. First and foremost, you must get whatever information is required to be able to participate actively and usefully in making decisions about your care. Second, each physician-specialist who participates in your care cannot escape responsibility for his or her own actions or for participating in decision making where appropriate. The physician-in-charge takes responsibility for the development of a plan of therapy, allows you to participate in decision making, sees to it that you have the information to do so, and coordinates the implementation of that plan.

In a nonteaching hospital, it is clear that your personal physician plays the quarterback role. Physicians in the hospital-based specialties or brought in as consultants should expect this and act accordingly.

In a teaching hospital, the situation is more complex. The resident assigned to you, your personal physician if you will, must fulfill the quarterback role. However, he or she must also recognize his or her obligation to use the experience of the supervising resident and attending physician to your benefit. He or she must recognize that the ultimate responsibility for the quality of medical care delivered by the resident team rests with the attending physician and supervising resident who are involved with the patient on a daily basis and who have an intimate knowledge of the patient's situation.

Does this mean that you should not ask anyone but your personal physician for information? Absolutely not. You have a right and a duty to prepare yourself as well as possible to participate in decisions about your care. At the same time, when asking information of a consultant or any physician involved in only one aspect of your care, you should remember that this physician is primarily concerned with one area of expertise and may only have information necessary for that particular part of your care. In view of this, it seems reasonable to ask consultants for explanations of procedures and descriptions of findings. However, you are less likely to get satisfactory responses to questions about what this means to the plan of therapy or how this affects the findings of another procedure or test. In other words, let the quarterback do the job of coordinating, but don't feel that the quarterback is the only physician from whom you may receive information.

Nurses

Good nursing is the key to a good hospital. The hospital's most important functions revolve around the nurse. If your doctor's plans for your care are to be implemented, it is largely up to nurses to see that this happens. Nurses are the ones who must see that medications are given, vital signs are taken, X-rays are done, tests are scheduled, and so on.

Just as importantly, it is the nurse who is responsible for observing and gathering information on your condition. Your doctor must rely on the nursing staff for these observations. This information must be accurate if appropriate decisions are to be made.

In short, it is the nurse who must take minute-to-minute and hour-to-hour responsibility for management of your medical care. But nursing is more than this. *Caring* for the patient as a human being is the oldest tradition in nursing. Knowing how to ease the burden of hospitalization and being willing to provide comfort to the patient are as basic to nursing as appropriate dispensing of medications or the accurate taking of vital signs.

Nursing is a tough job. The nurse must respond to requests and demands from patients, doctors, other hospital staff, friends and relatives of patients, and virtually anyone else who may have contact with you in the hospital. At the same time, nursing's own high standards must be met. Together these seem to produce a demand that the nurse be all things to all people and be perfect in the process. Finally, nursing is a physically demanding job. It requires considerable stamina to be on one's feet much of the time, move patients, and do whatever else is necessary for good patient care and still be ready to respond to the next demand for assistance.

To get the best out of your nurses, ask them to do what they do best. They are not maids or masseuses. Don't ask them to plump your pillow or rub your back or do anything that you can do for yourself. Don't assume that nurses bear all the responsibility for communicating with others, especially with your doctor. You still have a responsibility to participate in decisions about your medical care. Do expect them to carry out their professional obligation to see that the medical plans for therapy and observation are carried out. Finally, understand that they are subject to many demands. Be flexible where you can, but demand what you must have—excellence in professional nursing.

Support Personnel

It is easier to judge the quality of a hospital by the people who support the doctors and nurses than by looking at the doctors and nurses themselves. If the support staff is professional, responsive, and responsible, it suggests that the hospital has made a real effort to manage its activities effectively and efficiently. If the support staff appears uninterested and careless, the hospital—and its patients—will suffer.

Technicians

Almost every procedure in the hospital requires a technician. For example, do not be surprised if X-ray technicians take your X-rays completely on their own and if the radiologist looks only at the X-rays and not at you. This is the rule for basic X-rays of the chest, limbs, etc. Even when the radiologist is involved in the more complicated procedures, the quality of the X-rays and your experience with the procedure often depend on the X-ray technicians. Usually X-ray technicians are skilled and capable people, but they may not be in the habit of using protective shielding whenever possible. Do not hesitate to remind them.

If you require a blood test, do not be concerned that a doctor or nurse is not behind the needle. Obtaining a blood sample is a procedure in which those who do it the most often are most often the best at doing it. Since most hospitals now use laboratory technicians for this purpose, they are most likely to obtain an adequate sample with the least amount of trauma.

Dietician

A dietician will oversee the preparation of your meals, but you may not have any contact with this individual unless you require a special diet. Even if you don't require a special diet, don't miss an opportunity to talk with the dietician. Most often you will find them knowledgeable and informative as well as interested in your questions and concerns.

Orderlies   Orderlies are assigned to various sections of the hospital, including the operating room, the X-ray departments, and the wards. Their principal responsibilities are to get patients from place to place in the hospital and to perform the physically demanding tasks.

Remember, if you are interested in the quality of a hospital, check out the support staff. Their performance reflects that of the entire hospital.

8
The Hospital Routine

Your survival skill will receive a real test immediately upon admission to the hospital as you discover that you are "required" to sign an informed consent form (see Chapter 3) and undergo certain "routine" tests. These usually include a chest X-ray, blood tests, and a urinalysis. As indicated in Chapter 2, studies of these routine tests have failed to demonstrate their value or justify their risks. This is also true for the tests that are sometimes touted as routine prior to surgery.

The survivor's first rule for routine tests is clear:

UNDERGO NO TEST UNLESS THERE IS A CLEAR INDICATION FOR IT, AND "ROUTINE" IS NO INDICATION.

A second rule is also important:

IF TESTS ARE INDICATED FOR HOSPITAL ADMISSION OR FOR SURGERY, IT IS USUALLY BEST TO HAVE THESE DONE PRIOR TO ENTERING THE HOSPITAL (PRE-ADMISSION TESTING). THIS

CAN SAVE YOU MONEY AND SHORTEN YOUR HOSPITAL STAY.

Finally, as mentioned in Chapter 1:

ALMOST ALL TESTS CAN BE DONE WITHOUT ADMISSION TO THE HOSPITAL. TESTING ALONE IS USUALLY NOT A GOOD REASON FOR ADMISSION TO THE HOSPITAL.

Many tests done in the hospital are done early in the morning, prior to breakfast. There are two reasons for this:

1. Eating may affect the tests.
2. The laboratory or X-ray department must schedule the bulk of its workload in the morning so that it can handle urgent or emergency requests for tests.

Thus, the morning is the time of peak activity both on the wards where technicians are collecting blood samples and in the laboratory and X-ray departments themselves. The next busiest time is late in the afternoon when tests that are required twice daily are often performed.

Vital Signs and Physicians' Rounds

Vital Signs

Vital signs include checking the temperature, blood pressure, pulse, and respiratory rate. Virtually all patients have their vital signs checked at least once a day (in the morning); twice a day is not unusual; and for some patients, vital signs may be recorded three or more times per day. If the vital signs really need to be checked frequently, the patient is usually in an intensive care unit (ICU). Unlike most tests, even if the benefit of doing it one or more times a day is not obvious, there is very little risk in taking these measurements. Certainly, it's always a good thing to know your blood pressure, and it also ensures that you will make contact with the staff. If the taking of vital signs seems unnecessarily frequent, don't hesitate to discuss it with your physician.

Physicians' Rounds

Most physicians try to see their hospitalized patients at least twice a day although some patients can be managed effectively with a single visit. If you are on a teaching service, the residents will conduct rounds as a group in the morning and will check on patients individually during the rest of the day. The attending physician may accompany the residents on the morning rounds but is more likely to receive a report from the residents of the patients' conditions and then make separate rounds later in the day.

Drugs

Nothing is more rare than a patient in the hospital who is not taking medication. Sometimes, of course, the primary reason for hospitalization has been the need to administer medication in a particular way and closely observe its effects. But even when drugs are not necessary for therapy, it is routine to prescribe sleeping and pain medications. Laxatives are also a part of many physicians' "routine orders" for their hospitalized patients.

As explained in Chapter 2, drugs are a major part of the risk of hospitalization. Understanding the purpose of medications, how they are administered, and how you can increase the chances that they are used appropriately are essential survival skills.

Sleeping Pills

Being admitted to the hospital just about guarantees difficulty in sleeping. There are a variety of reasons for this:

- The hospital is noisy.
- Lights are left on a lot.
- You will have a stranger for a roommate.
- Other strangers (nurses, other hospital per-

sonnel, and your roommate's visitors) will continually come in and go out of the room unannounced.

Your roommate may be a saint, but it's almost a sure thing that your tastes in music and television programs will be different, your daily routines will have nothing in common, and at least one of you will snore. Not to mention that one or both of you just might be sick, meaning that discomfort will make sleep even more unlikely.

Your doctor knows this, and the order for a sleeping pill is the result. Most often this will be a minor tranquilizer such as Valium, Dalmane, or Halcion. These drugs are similar in terms of their chemical structures and, while some of them are promoted specifically as "hypnotics" (sleeping medications) rather than tranquilizers, there may be little practical difference in their effects. Current information suggests that certain tranquilizers may have an advantage in producing a more natural sleep, but this should not be regarded as proven beyond a reasonable doubt.

Some physicians will use drugs called antihistamines. These take advantage of the side effect of drowsiness, usually considered undesirable when antihistamines are used for other problems such as allergies.

Barbiturates and other older sedatives are seldom used today because they do not produce a natural sleep, they offer more risk with respect to side effects, and they are more strictly regulated because of their potential for abuse.

If you decide that the benefits of a sleeping medication outweigh the risks (discuss these with your doctor), you should ask that your doctor order them on a "PRN" basis. PRN means that you will receive the medication only if you request it, which should eliminate that classic affront to common sense, being awakened in order to be given a sleeping pill. Note that with some medicines and in some situations it is the nurse who will decide if the medication is needed when a PRN order is given. This should almost never be the case with sleeping pills. Make sure that you and your physician have a clear understanding as to how the PRN order will be interpreted, and remember that you *always* have the right to refuse any medication.

Pain Medicine

The relief of pain is one of the most basic objectives of medical care, and pain-relieving drugs represent major advances in medical science. Your doctor is likely to order a pain medication even if it is only acetaminophen to be used for a headache or other minor discomfort. Nevertheless, the appropriate use of pain medications requires that patient, doctor, and nurse work together. Here are some guidelines to facilitate this cooperation:

1. The patient is to decide whether the pain is mild, moderate, or severe. It behooves the doctor and nurse to respect this decision. At the same time, doctors and nurses cannot avoid their responsibility to make independent assessments of the degree of pain. But 99 percent of the time, the patient's estimate of the severity is the one that counts.

2. Matching the risks of the medication to the severity of the pain makes sense. Patients often underestimate the ability of oral pain relievers such as aspirin and acetaminophen to relieve pain. A request (or prescription) for a major pain medicine such as a narcotic for minor pain usually doesn't make sense.

3. At the same time, physicians and nurses should not overestimate the dangers of major pain relievers so that adequate pain relief is not achieved. The traditional "every four hours" schedule for pain medications has been demonstrated to be inadequate for pain relief in most cases of severe pain, simply because the medication wears off approximately three hours after it is administered.

4. As with all drugs, pain medicines have their risks and should be used only when needed. This means they should usually be ordered on a PRN basis.

The hallmarks of a good, cooperative effort with respect to pain medication are:

1. The physician orders a medication appropriate to the severity of pain.
2. The nurse administers the medication at an interval that provides adequate control of pain.
3. The patient uses the medication only when needed.

Intravenous (IV) and Intramuscular (IM) Injections

"IV" and "IM" are the medical jargon for two routes by which drugs may be administered: via the circulatory system (intravenous) or the muscles (intramuscular). IV administration has the advantage of providing the drug to the body in the quickest time, but it also means that the drug is more quickly cleared from the body. The result is that the intravenous route is used when it is necessary to administer medication quickly, to be sure that it is absorbed, or to attain higher concentrations in the body.

Laxatives

Exercise and adequate fiber in the diet are the best ways to promote bowel regularity. Avoiding constipation is another incentive to stay active in the hospital. If activity is restricted, a bulk or mild osmatic laxative (or a combination) such as Metamucil, Milk of Magnesia, or Haley's MO may be useful, but this should be only a temporary treatment.

The Surgical Routine

Surgeons, anaesthesiologists, and others who work in the operating room handle a large number of surgical procedures. Out of necessity, they have developed routines to make their system run smoothly. Because they are busy people, they may not remember that everything is new to you and that you may have questions about what is happening to you.

You will be instructed to have nothing to eat or drink on the morning of your operation. This is because it would be a dangerous situation if you were to vomit while under anaesthesia. Prior to surgery, hair may be shaved from the area to be operated on, and you will be dressed in a clean hospital gown to help reduce the risk of infection.

After surgery, you will be taken to a recovery room, where you will be monitored closely until you are ready to be transferred to your regular room. Some patients are surprised to find themselves hooked up to an IV or other tubes. Patients may have to be fed or receive fluids this way for a day or so following surgery. Sometimes tubes are used to drain off pus and other fluids.

Anaesthesia

There are two basic kinds of anaesthesia—general and local. Basically, general anaesthesia affects the entire system, bringing on an unconscious state. Local anaesthesia affects one area of the body—the part being operated on. With local anaesthesia, patients are aware of what's going on around them. There are advantages and disadvantages to both kinds of anaesthesia.

General anaesthesia is sometimes called gas, because it comes in a form that is inhaled. Among the common types used today are halothane and nitrous oxide (the dentist's laughing gas). Many patients like the idea of general anaesthesia, because it allows them to sleep through the procedure or because they find the thought of being stuck with needles in various parts of their body (as they would be when receiving a local anaesthetic) unpleasant.

The greatest drawback to general anaesthesia is that it carries a risk of coma or sudden death resulting from heart irregularities or collapse of the cardiovascular system. The reason for these serious reactions is not well understood, but anaesthesia is thought to be responsible for from 5 percent to 15 percent of all operative deaths.

A less severe drawback is the fact that people frequently experience severe nausea for several hours following general anaesthesia. And even though it comes in the form of a gas, it doesn't permit the squeamish to avoid needles. An IV is routinely inserted to begin the administration of drugs, and other injections may be given prior to surgery.

Local anaesthetics range from injections of drugs such as Novocain to numb a specific part of the body to substances that are injected into the spine to anaesthetize larger areas, for example, the pelvic region and legs.

The great advantage of a local anaesthetic, of course, is that it does not carry the risk of death associated with general anaesthesia. Local anaesthetics do not cause nausea, and they may actually provide better postoperative pain relief. However, while they do eliminate pain, they don't eliminate all sensation, and you may find that you are more aware than you'd like to be of what the surgeon is doing to you.

General anaesthesia is appropriate for many operations. For some operations, such as for hernias, local anaesthesia is the method of choice. Some procedures that were done almost exclusively under general anaesthesia in the past are now being done more frequently under local anaesthesia. An example of this is Caesarean section.

Surgeons often will decide to use general anaesthesia not because it is necessary, but because past experience has made them think that patients want and expect it. If you are interested in the possibility of using local anaesthesia, be sure to mention this to your surgeon.

A Word About Morning in the Hospital

As you can see, there is a whole lot going on in the morning. Doctors are making rounds on patients, blood samples are being drawn, vital signs are being taken, breakfast is being served, some patients are being whisked away to the X-ray department, and others are heading for surgery. Remember this if you are tempted to plan a morning activity that requires privacy and quiet, like sleeping. A hospital is not a boot camp; it just seems that way.

Diets

The fact that hospital food is notoriously unappetizing has little to do with medical restrictions placed on a patient's diet. It is more likely a result of mediocre preparation or because it was served while you were out for testing, etc., and was stone cold when you got back. General nutritional principles require that meals be balanced and not be prepared with salt. There is usually some choice in what you get to eat, and most patients are allowed to add salt if they like. If your food is cold, there is most likely a problem in getting the food to you. If your meal is unrecognizable, your physician may have ordered a special diet. Ask questions of your doctor, nurses, and food service staff, and complain when appropriate.

Smoking

The truth is that smoking has no place in the hospital. There is no place where there *should* be less tolerance for its toxic fumes. The presence of pure oxygen increases the fire hazard due to smoking as well. If you are a smoker, the opportunity to stop smoking can be the silver lining to your hospitalization cloud. Ask your doctor for help in dealing with the withdrawal; then enjoy your improved energy and health. If you are a nonsmoker, this is no time to be tolerant of things that make you sick. The hospital should provide a smoke-free environment without being asked to do so. If it has not, don't ask—demand it. Get your doctor to help if necessary.

9
Choosing Doctors and Hospitals

Carefully selecting a physician or surgeon is crucial to avoiding unnecessary hospitalization and surgery. Your choice of a hospital is important in determining how pleasant and how risky your stay will be. Since a doctor can practice in only a few hospitals, then choices go together; when you choose one, you are limiting your choices with respect to the other. This chapter will give you some guidelines for selecting doctors and hospitals.

Choosing a Doctor

Primary care physicians represent the initial contact between the patient and the medical establishment. They accept responsibility for the continued care of the patient and provide a wide variety of services. Primary care physicians are usually specialists in family practice, internal medicine, pediatrics, or obstetrics and gynecology.

If you go to a primary care physician with a problem, he or she will determine its nature and severity and recommend approaches to its solution. The primary care physician may suggest that you see a surgeon or other specialist.

In internal medicine, there is a specialty for nearly every organ system. Thus, cardiologists specialize in the heart; dermatologists, the skin; neurologists, the nervous system; nephrologists, the kidneys; and so forth. Within surgery, different types of operations have defined the specialties of particular surgeons. The ophthalmologist performs surgery on the eyes; the ear, nose, and throat (ENT) specialist on those areas; the thoracic surgeon on the chest; and the cardiac surgeon on the heart. The general surgeon operates in the abdominal cavity as well as other areas.

Doctors can practice alone or as part of a group. Some people prefer a doctor in solo practice because they like having one physician handling their case. Others prefer the involvement of more than one physician in their care and therefore like a group practice. You can receive good care in both arrangements, and this is purely a matter of personal preference. Seeing one doctor may mean that the two of you have more of an opportunity to get to know one another, and this is an important part of medical care to some people. However, no doctor is available 24 hours a day, and even the patients of a doctor in solo practice will at times need to see one of his or her colleagues.

If you need to find a doctor, you can begin by asking your friends. Question them closely about their experiences. Your county medical society can provide the names of physicians in your area who are accepting new patients. But remember, this is information, *not* a recommendation.

Asking doctors and nurses which doctors they use is a good idea. If you have a primary care physician, he or she can refer you to a surgeon or other specialist. You might want to ask medical professionals to recommend two or three doctors. If you ask a number of professionals, certain names will continue to show up. If there is a teaching hospital nearby, you can even call the chief resident in the specialty of interest (medicine, surgery, pediatrics, etc.) and ask for a recommendation. Chief residents usually have seen most of the good doctors at work and know who they are.

Some additional information can help you find a good surgeon. Competent surgeons will only be affiliated with accredited hospitals. They are likely to be certified by the American Board of Surgery. This means they have passed a rigorous test. If the initials F.A.C.S. follow the surgeon's name, this means that he or she is a fellow of the American College of Surgeons. This organization does no testing, but does require some evidence of dedication to excellence before conferring the title of fellow.* Of course, all of these criteria cannot guarantee a surgeon's competency, but they are good indicators.

A good surgeon will also perform a thorough examination prior to surgery. For example, before abdominal surgery this will include a rectal examination and a pelvic examination of women. Look for thoroughness in your surgeon.

Choosing a Hospital

Frequently, your choice of a hospital is determined by your choice of a doctor. It will be limited to those hospitals in which he or she practices. So you might want to investigate the hospitals in your area and use your preference as one of the factors that determines your choice of a doctor.

The general acute care hospital can be a highly sophisticated urban medical center or a 42-bed community hospital. You can get good care in both, but the nature of your problem may make one a better choice. For example, people needing

* Specialists in internal medicine, pediatrics, and obstetrics and gynecology can also be fellows of professional organizations limited to their specialties. Therefore, "fellowship" can be one of the criteria you use for selecting a primary care physician as well.

open-heart surgery would be much better off in a large hospital center that is staffed and equipped to handle their needs. An individual experiencing complications in the treatment of diabetes, arthritis, or another chronic disease can receive adequate care in a smaller hospital that might be more conveniently located.

Some hospitals are teaching hospitals, which means they are involved in training physicians through an affiliation with a medical school. You will probably receive good care in a teaching hospital, but you may find the number of people involved in your care disconcerting. Chapter 7 contains an explanation of the staffing arrangements in a teaching hospital.

It was mentioned earlier that competent surgeons are affiliated only with accredited hospitals. The Joint Commission on Accreditation of Hospitals makes inspections and certifies that surgery and other medical procedures are done according to their standards. You can find out whether a hospital is accredited by asking your doctor or calling the hospital. **It is very important that the hospital you use be accredited.**

If you have had prior experience with a hospital, you probably noticed whether the facilities were clean and well maintained, and whether the nursing and support staff seemed competent and happy. A well-cared-for facility and satisfied, good quality employees are indicators of a good hospital.

Selecting good doctors and hospitals is important, but it does not take away the patient's obligation to understand what is happening throughout treatment. Remember to stay informed every step of the way, to undergo no unnecessary tests or procedures, and to stay out of the hospital if you can.

Part IV

SURGICAL ADMISSIONS

If you require surgery for a life-threatening condition such as a ruptured spleen, you do not face a choice. If the surgery is not performed, you face imminent death.

But usually the patient has a choice to make about having surgery done; although in some cases, choosing not to have surgery is foolish. Just about any operation that is not performed in an emergency, life-or-death situation is considered *elective surgery*.

Anyone facing a decision about surgery must be aware of all available treatment options, including that of not having it done. It is also important to know what kind of results it is realistic to expect. Frequently, these decisions are subjective—*you* must decide whether the relief of discomfort outweighs the risks of surgery. The chapters in this part of the book are designed to provide guidance in making decisions about the kinds of elective surgery most commonly performed.

Providing specific information on every kind of elective surgery in a book like this would have been impossible. But we have provided basic guidelines to follow in deciding about any kind of operation: specifically, getting a second opinion, inquiring about treatment alternatives, and weighing the benefits and risks. The same guidelines apply to cosmetic surgery as well, but in this case individuals face a very personal decision—whether feeling good about their appearance is worth the risks of surgery.

10
Hernia

To surgeons, a hernia operation is the fundamental surgical procedure. It is the operation that general surgeons will perform most frequently. Surgical training is even measured in "hernia equivalents," a term that bears testimony to this procedure's position as the basic unit of surgical experience. If you should find yourself on the business end of a surgeon's scalpel, there is a good chance that a hernia is the reason.

A hernia is a protrusion or bulging of a body tissue through the structure that contains it. There are many medical terms that contain the term hernia—inguinal hernia, umbilical hernia, hiatal hernia, herniated disc, etc. However, when the word hernia is used alone, it refers to *inguinal hernia*. An inguinal hernia is a bulging through a weak portion of the abdominal wall in the groin area. If large enough, such a bulging may allow an abdominal organ, usually the small intestine, to slip out of the abdomen into the hernia sac. Most of the time the organ is able to slip out of the hernia sac and back into the abdomen. When it is trapped in the hernia sac, as sometimes happens, physicians refer to this as an *incarcerated hernia*. If the organ is trapped in such a

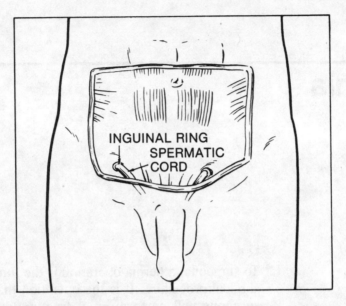

The inguinal canal is the tube through which a testis descends into the scrotum. This usually happens just before birth.

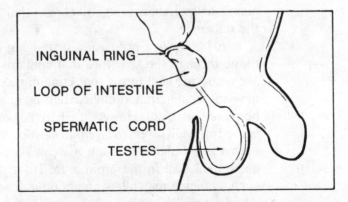

In one kind of inguinal hernia, part of an abdominal organ passes through the inguinal canal.

way that the blood supply to the organ is shut off, then it is termed a *strangulated hernia*.

Inguinal hernias account for about 90 percent of the hernias seen by physicians. *Umbilical hernias* (a bulging around the umbilicus or belly button, usually seen in children) account for more than 5 percent of total hernias; *femoral hernias* (a bulging also in the groin area but lower than inguinal hernias) comprise about 2 percent. All other hernias of the abdominal wall—and there are more than 15 different kinds—account for the remaining percentage.

This discussion is concerned principally with inguinal hernias, although femoral hernias require essentially the same considerations. Umbilical hernias in children are also discussed.

Local vs. General Anaesthesia

Although hernia operations traditionally have been done under general anaesthesia, the consensus among surgeons doing research in this field is that procedures done under local anaesthesia have great advantages.

1. The risk of death and complications seems to be lower, perhaps less than half of that when general anaesthesia is used.
2. Because the patient is awake (although drowsy) and can cooperate, the strength of the hernia repair can be tested during the procedure rather than waiting to see if it holds together after the patient wakes up.
3. Most patients are able to walk without discomfort within several hours of finishing the procedure. More than 85 percent who have hernia operations using local anaesthesia go home on the day of the operation; more than 90 percent go home within 24 hours of the operation. So there seems to be a real savings in terms of time, money, and discomfort.

Local anaesthesia is for elective, uncomplicated procedures. General anaesthesia is the rule
if the hernia is incarcerated and if there is any
evidence of strangulation.

Some patients request general anaesthesia
thinking that it is better to "sleep" through the
procedure and thus avoid discomfort and worry.
Interestingly, it appears to be the consensus of
both surgeons and patients that the discomfort of
the local anaesthesia approach is much less than
that of general anaesthesia. Some surgeons believe
that local anaesthesia has a residual effect that
minimizes discomfort eight to 48 hours after surgery: This is when patients having general anaesthesia usually experience considerable difficulty.

Alternatives to Hernia Surgery

The alternatives to surgery for a hernia are to do
nothing or wear a truss (a pad attached to a belt and
held in place by straps or a spring). Few subjects
elicit less enthusiasm among surgeons than
trusses. Although the truss is designed to prevent
the return of a hernia, surgeons almost always
describe it as an ill-fitting, uncomfortable, and
ineffective device. An article arguing for the truss
as the treatment of choice has not appeared in the
medical literature since 1947. In any event, there
are no modern scientific studies of the value of
trusses in relieving discomfort or preventing incar-
ceration of hernias.

Doing nothing has not been studied either.
The chance of a hernia becoming incarcerated in
any one year appears to be less than 0.3 percent.
Nothing in the scientific literature suggests how
often the discomfort will disappear on its own or
get worse. So, it seems reasonable to assume that
it will stay about the same.

Benefits

There are two reasons for elective hernia operations:

1. To relieve discomfort

2. To avoid the possibility of a strangulated hernia.

Patients tend to emphasize the former while physicians focus on the latter. The effectiveness of a hernia operation in relieving discomfort has not been studied in a rigorous scientific fashion, perhaps because physicians do not think that it is an important reason for doing the operation. This is too bad, since a close examination of the risks and benefits of elective hernia operations suggests that **relief of discomfort is usually the primary benefit of the operation, not its ability to prevent strangulated hernias.**

Not that strangulated hernias are to be regarded lightly. Emergency surgery for a strangulated hernia is associated with a risk of death that may be as high as 10 to 40 times the risk of death associated with an elective hernia operation. There is no question that the emergency operation is more risky than the elective one. But the critical question is how likely one is to have a strangulated hernia (and, therefore, an emergency operation) if one does not have the elective operation. As stated above, one study suggested that less than 0.3 percent of individuals with inguinal hernias who did not have an operation would develop a strangulated hernia in any given year. Since the chance of needing an emergency operation is so small, the value of attempting to prevent that chance must also be small.

Hernias in Children

There has been no formal analysis of the risks versus the benefits with respect to operating on inguinal hernias in children. However, it appears that the risk of a lifetime of living with a hernia is greater and the risk of the procedure is less in children than it is in adults. In addition, the operative procedure itself is somewhat more simple in children. If a hernia is detected on one side in a child, there is about a 50–50 chance that there is a hernia present but undetected on the other side.

For this reason, it is not uncommon for the surgeon to explore the other side when repairing the hernia that has been detected. Finally, even though general anaesthesia is the rule, children almost always go home a few hours after this procedure is completed. Thus, almost all children's hernia operations are done on an ambulatory basis.

In summary, we lack the type of analysis on children's hernia operations that has been done on adult hernia operations. Because the procedure is somewhat more simple, it can be done on an ambulatory basis. Also, since the risk of a lifetime of living with a hernia seems to be somewhat greater, virtually all inguinal hernias in children are operated on.

Umbilical Hernias

These bulgings around the belly button are frequent and occur more commonly in black children (as many as one-third of black children will have an umbilical hernia at birth). Most of these hernias resolve themselves without treatment of any kind. Surgical repair is reserved for those hernias that remain large at the age of two to three. Small hernias may continue to be watched. In other words, it is rare to operate on an umbilical hernia.

Risks

The risk of death for the first elective hernia operation in adults has been estimated to be as low as 0.1 percent and as high as 2.3 percent. It is important to note that many of these operations were done with general anaesthesia, which appears to be considerably more risky than local anaesthesia (see page 73). A reasonable estimate is in the neighborhood of 0.2 percent.

We said "first elective hernia operation" because there is a chance that the hernia will recur, requiring another operation. In fact, it is possible that it will recur several times and require several operations. Studies have reported first recurrence rates from 1 percent to 30 percent; the current consensus seems to be about 10 percent. Second recurrences apparently have a higher probability. This means that once you have had one recurrence, there is about a 30 percent chance that you'll have another. The risks of operations to correct these recurrences must be counted in figuring the risks of elective surgery for hernias.

There are, of course, complications associated with hernia operations that do not result in death, such as infections and the complications of anaesthesia. Complications that require an extended hospital stay or further surgery appear to occur in about 1 percent of cases.

Costs

Optimally, hernia operations should be done on an ambulatory basis. It is interesting to note, though, that the average hospital stay for hernia surgery is four days. This average includes cases in which there were complications and those in which the patient was "routinely" admitted to the hospital for several days.

The cost of this surgery will probably be about $900 for ambulatory surgery and from $2,000 to $4,000 for surgery with hospitalization of four days. However, the cost of medical care varies considerably from one region of the country to another, and your final bill could be above or below this range.

Making Decisions About Hernias

Ideally, one might make a choice using a technique called *decision analysis*. With this method, the outcome of having an elective operation would be weighed against the outcome associated with not having the operation. The "no surgery" side would include the probability of strangulation occurring followed by the probability of death. The "surgery" side would include a consideration of the probability of death due to the first operation, the probability of recurrences, and the probability of death due to operations for recurrences. Such an analysis has been conducted by researchers at Harvard, and their conclusion is as follows:

1. The risk of death is small regardless of whether or not surgery is performed.
2. However, the risk of death actually appears to be somewhat greater if one has the operation than if one does not.

There are some important things to note about this conclusion.

First, the estimate of the risk of death depends on age as well as probabilities chosen for the analysis. The principal author of this particular study felt that the most reasonable estimate for a 65-year-old man was that the risk of death was 5½ times greater with an operation than without one. Using different assumptions, the risk of death becomes almost the same with or without the operation. However, under no set of circumstances did it appear that the risk of death was increased if an individual did not have an operation.

Second, the risks of the operation included procedures done under general anaesthesia, which appears to increase the danger of the operation. Operations done under local anaesthesia do not appear to have the same risk. (See page 73.)

The bottom line is this: A hernia operation should not be done out of fear of death due to an incarcerated or strangulated hernia.

To summarize, more important considerations include:

- The risk of death may be no different with or without surgery.
- The amount of discomfort that the hernia gives and the capability of the operation to relieve that discomfort should be considered.
- If you decide to have the operation, having it done under local anaesthesia usually means that there will be less risk for you. There will be much less cost,

and you can go in, have the operation, and leave all in the same day.

- Although the current rule is to operate on virtually all inguinal hernias in children, you still should discuss the risks and benefits of the procedure with the surgeon and make a decision using the best available information. Remember that this should be done on an ambulatory basis unless it is a complicated situation.

Hernia

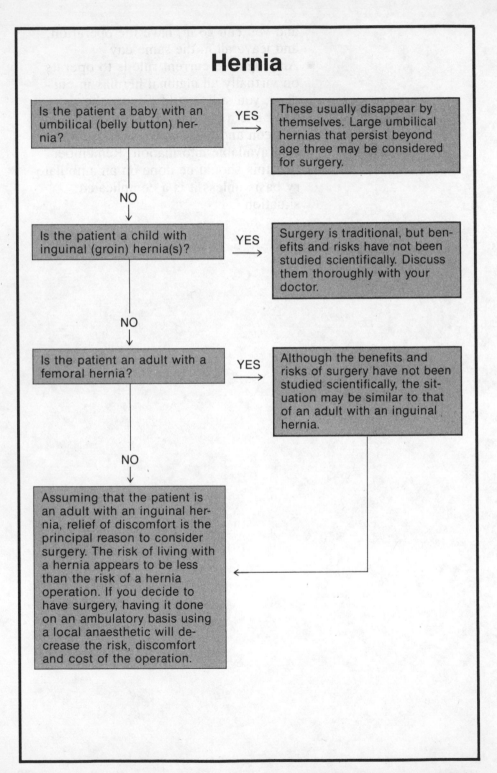

Is the patient a baby with an umbilical (belly button) hernia?

YES → These usually disappear by themselves. Large umbilical hernias that persist beyond age three may be considered for surgery.

NO ↓

Is the patient a child with inguinal (groin) hernia(s)?

YES → Surgery is traditional, but benefits and risks have not been studied scientifically. Discuss them thoroughly with your doctor.

NO ↓

Is the patient an adult with a femoral hernia?

YES → Although the benefits and risks of surgery have not been studied scientifically, the situation may be similar to that of an adult with an inguinal hernia.

NO ↓

Assuming that the patient is an adult with an inguinal hernia, relief of discomfort is the principal reason to consider surgery. The risk of living with a hernia appears to be less than the risk of a hernia operation. If you decide to have surgery, having it done on an ambulatory basis using a local anaesthetic will decrease the risk, discomfort and cost of the operation.

11

Tonsillectomy and Adenoidectomy

Surgery to remove the tonsils (tonsillectomy) and surgery to remove the adenoids (adenoidectomy) were performed together so often in the past that they generally were regarded as a single procedure referred to simply as "T&A." Today they are more likely to be thought of as separate procedures, as they should be. Still, separately or combined, these procedures are by far the most frequent operations performed on American children. It is estimated that approximately 600,000 are done each year, down from approximately 1,200,000 in 1965.

The major reason for the decline in the number of operations is the realization by both doctors and parents that they are often unnecessary. In the past, frequent sore throats or frequent ear infections were the reasons most often given for doing a T&A. It is now known that tonsillectomy is of little or no value with respect to sore throats, and that usually there are safer, less costly alternatives to adenoidectomy for frequent ear infections.

The tonsils and adenoids are composed of lymphoid tissue—the kind of tissue that makes antibodies and is important in developing immunity. The exact role of tonsils and adenoids remains myste-

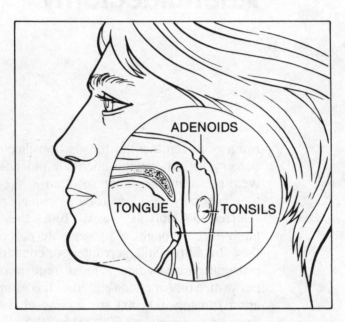

The tonsils and adenoids are collections of lymphoid tissue located at the back of the throat and at the back of the nose.

rious, but it is clear that they are in the way of almost everything swallowed or breathed, so they often receive first exposure to bacteria, viruses, and other substances with which the body comes in contact. For this reason, many physicians believe that the tonsils and the adenoids help us develop immunity to these potentially harmful organisms and substances. There is some evidence indicating that this might be the case; for example, the amount of antibody against the polio virus decreases after a tonsillectomy and adenoidectomy, and the risk of polio increases after the operation.

The size of the tonsils and adenoids increases up to the age of six or seven and then gradually decreases. Thus, it is quite possible that a younger child will have larger tonsils than an older brother or sister or an adult.

These operations are simple in concept. The tissue is cut away from the sides of the throat using a thin wire loop or a scalpel. If there are no complications, the patient can return home after recovery from the anaesthesia, and an overnight stay in the hospital is not necessary.

Benefits

Tonsillectomy and adenoidectomy are separate surgical procedures and should be considered separately; automatically thinking in terms of T&A has led to unnecessary procedures.

The tonsils and/or adenoids can become so enlarged that they interfere with breathing and/or swallowing. In rare cases the interference with breathing is so severe that it strains the heart and lungs and can even lead to heart damage. If the obstruction is severe, a tonsillectomy and/or adenoidectomy should be considered.

Enlargement of the adenoids may block the Eustachian tube, the passage that leads from the ear to the throat. This causes fluid to accumulate in the ear. Recurrent ear infections may occur if the blockage persists for a long period. An adenoidectomy can relieve this blockage and probably decreases the number of ear infections. However, it is easier and safer to relieve the blockage by making a small hole in the eardrum (myringotomy). Usually a small tube is placed in the hole to keep it open and promote drainage.

Very large adenoids may also block nasal passages and interfere in the development of normal speech. Although an adenoidectomy can help in these unusual cases, there are certain specific instances when it should *not* be done. Specifically, when function of the palate (roof of the mouth) is not normal, an adenoidectomy can be disastrous to the child's speech. Careful examination of the palate and special X-rays can help in making this decision. The presence of tumors in the tonsils or the threat of recurrent tonsillar abscesses are also unusual reasons for having a tonsillectomy or adenoidectomy performed.

Frequent sore throats are not an accepted reason for surgery. The proposal of surgery for this problem should be regarded with the utmost suspicion. Do not consider such a proposal seriously unless several other physicians agree that this is a unique instance when a sore throat is a valid indication for operating. We are not convinced that such a situation can occur.

Risks

The principal hazards of T&As are the risks due to hemorrhage, which increase with age, and the risks due to anaesthesia, which decrease with age. The risk of death has been estimated to be as high as one in 1,000. The risk of a serious complication (hemorrhage, infection) is probably the same.

Costs

If T&A surgery is to be performed at all, it should be on an ambulatory basis. However, the average stay for removal of the tonsils and adenoids in 1984 was about two days. This average includes cases in which there were complications and those in which the patient was "routinely" admitted to the hospital for several days.

The cost of this surgery will probably be about $900 for ambulatory surgery and between $1,500 and $3,000 for surgery with hospitalization. However, the cost of medical care varies considerably from one region of the country to another, and your bill could wind up either above or below this range.

Making Decisions About Tonsillectomy and Adenoidectomy

The valid reasons for tonsillectomy and/or adenoidectomy are indicated in the flow chart on page 86 and discussed above. In summary, there are times when obstruction by tonsils and/or adenoids is so great that it interferes with breathing, swallowing, or normal speech development. There may be times when blockage of the Eustachian tube cannot be relieved by a myringotomy and will require an adenoidectomy. There will only be a few operations required because of tumors or tonsillar abscesses. Even if all of these reasons for surgery were put together, they could not possibly justify even a tiny fraction of the 600,000 operations performed each year. It seems clear that most operations are still being done to "cure" frequent sore throats and/or frequent ear problems. It is equally clear that the risks far outweigh the benefits in such cases.

The indications for tonsillectomy and/or adenoidectomy have been so abused that a second opinion is appropriate any time that one of these procedures is suggested.

If it should be determined that surgery is appropriate and necessary, having the procedure done on an ambulatory basis will reduce the risks and costs in most instances.

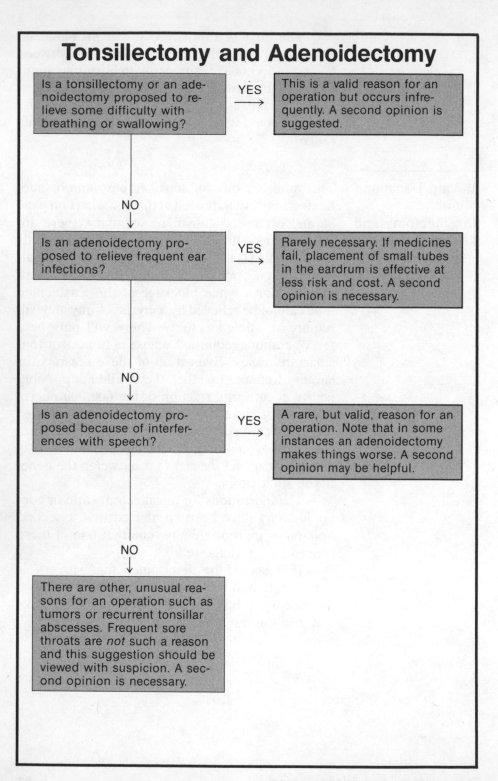

Tonsillectomy and Adenoidectomy

Is a tonsillectomy or an adenoidectomy proposed to relieve some difficulty with breathing or swallowing?

→ YES → This is a valid reason for an operation but occurs infrequently. A second opinion is suggested.

NO ↓

Is an adenoidectomy proposed to relieve frequent ear infections?

→ YES → Rarely necessary. If medicines fail, placement of small tubes in the eardrum is effective at less risk and cost. A second opinion is necessary.

NO ↓

Is an adenoidectomy proposed because of interferences with speech?

→ YES → A rare, but valid, reason for an operation. Note that in some instances an adenoidectomy makes things worse. A second opinion may be helpful.

NO ↓

There are other, unusual reasons for an operation such as tumors or recurrent tonsillar abscesses. Frequent sore throats are *not* such a reason and this suggestion should be viewed with suspicion. A second opinion is necessary.

12

Gallbladder Operations

The gallbladder stores bile, a mixture of substances produced by the liver, which aids in the digestion of food. The gallbladder empties bile into the intestine in response to eating a meal. While this seems to be a most helpful arrangement, you can do perfectly well without your gallbladder. This seemingly optional organ can cause real problems when portions of the bile solidify to form gallstones.

Gallbladder Diseases/Disorders

Gallstones

Almost all of the problems of the gallbladder are associated with gallstones. It appears that most gallstones form because the liver secretes an abnormal (lithogenic) bile that contains too much cholesterol in proportion to the other chemicals present, bile salts and phospholipids. While diet influences the composition of bile, it does not appear that diet alone can cause or prevent gallstones in most people. It is more likely that the major factor in determining the risk of gallstones is a genetic predisposition. For example, in certain American Indian tribes, almost

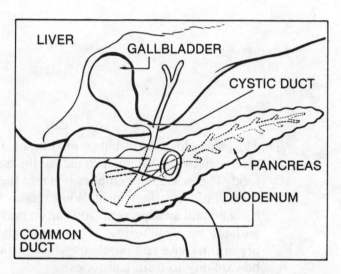

LIVER

GALLBLADDER

CYSTIC DUCT

PANCREAS

DUODENUM

COMMON DUCT

The gallbladder empties bile, which aids in the digestion of food, into the intestine. Bile passes from the gallbladder, through the cystic duct, and into the common duct, the tube that carries the secretions of the pancreas, liver and gall-bladder to the intestine.

all of the women and many of the men over age 30 have so-called lithogenic bile.

Before the age of 50, women are about three times as likely to have gallstones as men. It has been estimated that approximately 18 million women and 6 million men in the United States have gallstones. After the age of 50, the difference between men and women becomes progressively smaller. Exactly how many people actually have gallstones is not known since most gallstones are never detected, and the vast majority of people who have them never know it.

Several years ago, there was hope that a drug called chenodeoxycholoc acid would dissolve gallstones and sharply reduce the need for surgery. However, the research now suggests that it works in only one of seven persons with gallstones and causes a distinct rise in the cholesterol level of the blood. There is also the risk of liver damage with the treatment. For these reasons, the drug is rarely recommended.

Cancer of the Gallbladder

Cancer of the gallbladder is a relatively uncommon tumor that occurs most often in older women. While cancer of the gallbladder is usually associated with gallstones, it has not been demonstrated that gallstones *cause* cancer of the gallbladder. However, because of the association between gallstones and cancer of the gallbladder, it has been argued that the gallbladder should be removed if gallstones are discovered even if they cause no symptoms.

The research currently available does not settle this argument conclusively. Although there are studies that suggest some benefit if these "silent" gallstones are removed, fear of cancer alone does not appear to be a compelling reason for surgery. Most physicians do not press for an operation when gallstones are discovered in the course of investigating another problem.

Acute Cholecystitis   Acute cholecystitis is the medical term for a gall-bladder attack. Pain and tenderness in the right upper portion of the abdomen are the most important and consistent symptoms of acute cholecystitis. Sometimes the pain is brought on by a meal, and in some cases it may be relieved by vomiting. However, this is not always true. More than 90 percent of the time, acute cholecystitis occurs when a gallstone blocks the cystic duct (the tube that allows bile to leave the gallbladder). This causes swelling, may diminish blood supply to the gallbladder, and creates a situation in which infection with bacteria is more likely to occur. When acute cholecystitis is not associated with gallstones, it usually follows some injury, including surgery; this injury does not necessarily have to be to the gallbladder itself or even to the abdomen.

Special X-rays (cholangiograms) are the most important tests for determining whether the pain is due to cholecystitis, but other tests, including electrocardiograms and blood tests, are usually necessary in order to give the most accurate diagnosis.

Gallbladder Surgery   "Gallbladder operation" almost always means complete removal of the gallbladder (cholecystectomy). Since the human body doesn't absolutely require the gallbladder, the simplest and most satisfactory approach is to remove it entirely.

Occasionally, the gallbladder is so devitalized (necrotic) and close to falling apart that removal will not be attempted and a procedure that allows drainage of the gallbladder (cholecystostomy) will be performed instead. Cholecystectomy is usually done at a later date.

Cholecystectomy may be accompanied by another procedure called a *common duct explora-*

tion. The common duct is the tube that collects the secretions of the pancreas, liver, and gallbladder and delivers them to the intestine. (The cystic duct leads from the gallbladder to the common duct. See illustration on page 88.) If there are signs that the common duct may be blocked by a gallstone, the surgeon may do exploratory surgery in an effort to find the gallstone and remove it. This procedure substantially increases the difficulty of the operation as well as the recovery time. Whether or not the common duct is explored is the most important factor in determining how ill you feel and how long you must stay in the hospital following the operation.

Benefits

About 75 percent of patients with acute cholecystitis will lose all of their symptoms within one to four days of the beginning of the attack even if treatment consists only of bed rest, pain relievers, and adequate fluid intake. The remaining 25 percent will have a progressively toxic course requiring hospitalization; emergency surgery is often necessary. Unfortunately, those patients who recover completely without hospitalization or surgery have about a 50 percent chance of having another attack within ten years *if* gallstones are present after recovery. However, if there are no gallstones, the chance of another attack appears to be much less than 50 percent, perhaps no greater than for any other person without gallstones. The situation in which repeated attacks occur may be referred to as *chronic cholecystitis* or *recurrent cholecystitis*. Surgery has become the treatment of choice for cholecystitis because medical and dietary treatments cannot protect against these recurring attacks.

Risks

As with many operations, the risk of complications and death is less when the procedure can be done on an elective rather than an emergency basis. In the case of a cholecystectomy for acute cholecystitis, it is important to note that a cholecystectomy done soon after the diagnosis is made does *not* mean that this is an emergency operation. An emergency operation is one that is done as quickly as possible because there is no alternative, i.e., without the operation death or severe disability seems certain or at least very likely.

The risk of death for an elective cholecystectomy has been estimated to be approximately 0.1 percent to 0.3 percent; risk of death for an emergency cholecystectomy may be as high as 5 percent. The risk of major complications (infection, pancreatitis) are approximately the same.

Costs

The optimal length of stay for cholecystectomy is two to three days. An additional day should be added if surgery includes a common duct exploration. However, the average length of stay for gallbladder surgery is nine days. This average includes cases in which there were complications and those in which the patient was "routinely" admitted to the hospital for several days.

The cost of gallbladder surgery will probably range between $1,900 and $3,000. However, the cost of medical care varies considerably from one region of the country to another, and your final bill could be above or below this range.

Making Decisions About Gallbladder Surgery

The flowchart on page 95 illustrates the main points in making decisions about gallbladder operations.

If you have a clear-cut case of acute cholecystitis, surgery is usually recommended to prevent the disease from progressing to a toxic stage and prevent recurrences. In addition to the discomfort involved, each recurrence carries with it the chance of developing into a toxic state requiring emergency surgery with its increased risk of complication and death.

There is controversy as to when the surgery should be performed. Since most acute attacks will resolve on their own, some surgeons prefer to wait until this occurs and perform the surgery as an elective procedure. However, the majority of medical opinion now appears to favor immediate operation on the basis that this prevents progression of the disease and, on the average, reduces morbidity and mortality. Again, the research currently available does not allow this controversy to be settled once and for all. At present, the best advice appears to be that you should have the operation without delay if the diagnosis is made with a high degree of certainty.

If you should elect to "ride out" a first gallbladder attack, then you must take into account the chance of further attacks as discussed previously. If gallstones are still present, most physicians will advise you to consider surgery. If there are none, then the usual advice is to "wait and see."

In summary, if you definitely have acute cholecystitis, then early surgery is the choice most recommended. But if the attack passes without surgery *and* there are no remaining gallstones, observation rather than elective surgery is the rule.

The question of what to do with "silent" gallstones is also somewhat controversial. Such gallstones are usually discovered when an X-ray is done in the course of investigating some problem other than gallbladder disease. The best information suggests that less than 20 percent of the people with silent gallstones will eventually develop symptoms of gallbladder disease. Nevertheless, the possibility of symptoms and the association of gallstones with cancer of the gallbladder pose a question worth considering: Do the risks of these problems outweigh the risks of the operation? Most physicians will discuss the available information with you but will suggest watching and waiting rather than surgery.

Finally, there are situations in which the diagnosis of cholecystitis is possible or even probable but not certain. In this situation, it may well be best to wait and see since an operation is especially undesirable in the presence of some of the diseases that can mimic cholecystitis, i.e., inflammation of the pancreas (pancreatitis) and heart attack. However, recurrence of the problem and the presence of gallstones will favor surgery. A diagnosis of "possible" or "probable" cholecystitis is one of those times, all too common in medicine, when there is considerable risk regardless of what is done. In general, the best advice is to delay as long as is prudent while attempting to increase the certainty of the diagnosis.

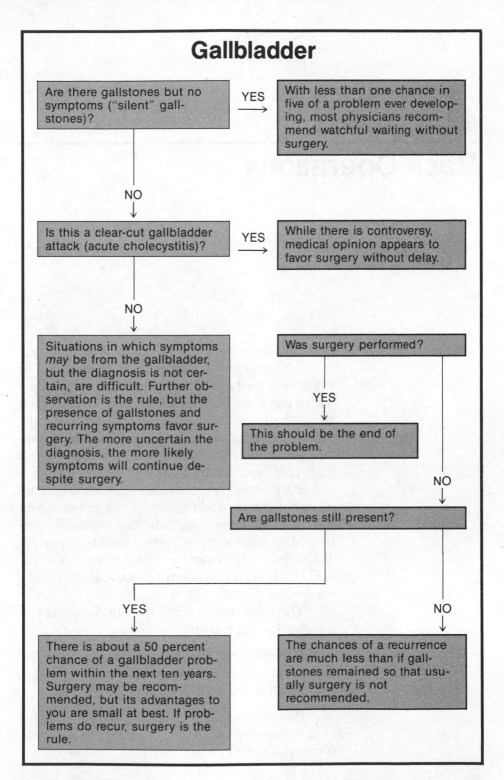

Gallbladder

Are there gallstones but no symptoms ("silent" gallstones)? — YES → With less than one chance in five of a problem ever developing, most physicians recommend watchful waiting without surgery.

NO ↓

Is this a clear-cut gallbladder attack (acute cholecystitis)? — YES → While there is controversy, medical opinion appears to favor surgery without delay.

NO ↓

Situations in which symptoms *may* be from the gallbladder, but the diagnosis is not certain, are difficult. Further observation is the rule, but the presence of gallstones and recurring symptoms favor surgery. The more uncertain the diagnosis, the more likely symptoms will continue despite surgery.

Was surgery performed?

YES ↓

This should be the end of the problem.

NO ↓

Are gallstones still present?

YES ↓

There is about a 50 percent chance of a gallbladder problem within the next ten years. Surgery may be recommended, but its advantages to you are small at best. If problems do recur, surgery is the rule.

NO ↓

The chances of a recurrence are much less than if gallstones remained so that usually surgery is not recommended.

13

Back Operations

Few problems are more common than low back pain. It is estimated that more than 70 percent of us will have at least one episode of back pain some time during our lives. Fortunately, surgery for back pain should be a relatively infrequent occurrence. One expert has suggested that surgery can be recommended for only 2 percent of those people whose back pain is so severe that they are referred to a university hospital for evaluation. Such referrals account for only a tiny fraction of the persons with back pain. However, back surgery is actually performed far more frequently than would be expected. This is probably because of differences in how patients and physicians interpret the reasons for the operations.

There are two principal reasons for doing surgery for low back pain:

1. To relieve pressure on a nerve
2. As a last resort when pain continues and all other therapies have failed.

Pressure on the nerve usually occurs when one of the discs that separates the bones in the back (vertebral discs) bulges out and presses on the

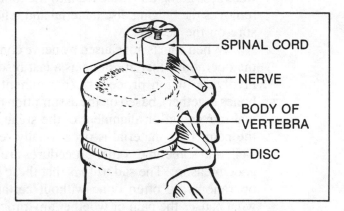

The vertebrae, or separate bones of the back, are separated by flexible flattened discs.

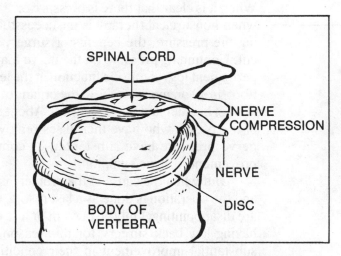

When the back is strained, one of the discs can bulge out and press on nerves as they leave the spinal cord.

nerves as they leave the spinal cord. This is the infamous herniated or slipped disc, which may cause back pain as well as sciatica (pain, numbness, and/or weakness going down the leg into the foot). Surgery removes the bulging disc material and relieves pressure on the nerves.

When pain is not caused by nerve compression, the operations that are done as a last resort usually involve a fusion procedure (permanently joining bones together), based on the assumption that abnormal movement or alignment of the spine is causing the pain. Disc material is occasionally removed as well, and sometimes other procedures are added for good measure. The sad truth is that these last-resort operations are often done without certainty as to what causes the pain or whether any procedure will help. There is a tendency to do whatever might help and hope for the best.

Benefits

When it is clear that there is pressure on a nerve and when nonsurgical therapy is unsuccessful in relieving the pressure, the benefits of surgery are clear-cut. Continuing pressure on the nerve may result in permanent loss of muscle function in the leg and foot (foot drop) or, more rarely, in the organs of the pelvis (loss of bladder and bowel control). About 80 percent of the people who have their discs removed due to nerve pressure have substantial or complete improvement in their symptoms.

But when the cause of the problem is not clear, and the operation is done as a last resort, the results are disappointing. Only 50 percent or less of persons having low back surgery for this reason will have substantial improvement in their condition. However, a relief rate of 40 percent or more could be expected from a placebo effect on the basis of studies concerning other types of severe pain. In other words, the relief rate appears to be not much better than would be expected from the psychological effect of having surgery alone.

Part IV: Surgical Admissions

Risks

Operations on the back are major surgical procedures involving the risks of anaesthesia, damage to nerves or the spinal cord, and infection. In addition, they are particularly likely to increase the risk of inactivity since bed rest may be prolonged after many of the procedures. Death rates for the operation have been estimated at between 0.1 percent and 1 percent.

Costs

With all back surgery, the sooner you can be up and moving around, the better. The optimal length of stay for surgical removal of a disc is two days; for a fusion procedure, it is four days. Many people spend a long time in the hospital after back surgery—the average length of stay is 12 days. This average does include cases in which there were complications. But it also includes patients who were "routinely" admitted to the hospital for several days.

The cost of back surgery can range between $3,000 and $12,000 or even more. However, the cost of medical care varies considerably from one region of the country to another, and your bill could wind up either above or below this range.

Making Decisions About Back Surgery

The major benefit of back surgery is the prevention of permanent damage caused by pressure on a nerve. However, most often pressure on a nerve can be relieved without surgery. Thus, a disc operation makes sense only when the back problems are substantial and when nonsurgical therapy has failed.

The most difficult part of this decision is determining when to give up on nonsurgical therapy. Most back specialists will not even do the test necessary for considering surgery (myelogram) until nonsurgical therapy has been tried for several months. However, in cases with severe and progressive loss of nerve function as evidenced by loss of muscular control, surgery may be appropriate much sooner, even within a matter of days of onset of the problem. Such rapid progression is rare, fortunately.

Back surgery done as a last resort is much more difficult to justify. Even when the operation provides relief, this often proves to be temporary. The simple truth is that surgery is not a solution for the vast majority of people with chronic back pain. Certainly, surgery seems an unwise choice unless nonsurgical methods have been used appropriately and conscientiously, and unless the physicians recommending the procedure can be specific as to what will be done and why it will help. To give yourself the best chance at success, get a recommendation from more than one physician. At least one of the physicians recommending the surgery should be a nonsurgical specialist in back pain, usually in the subspecialty of internal medicine called rheumatology.

Be sure that all facets of nonsurgical therapy have been explored before you agree to an operation.

Back Operations

Is the operation suggested because of pressure on a nerve?	YES →	Surgery is appropriate IF: 1. There is significant pain or loss of muscle control. 2. The cause of the pressure is clearly identified in the back. 3. Nonsurgical therapy does not bring relief.

NO ↓

Is the operation suggested because of prolonged or severe back pain but without evidence of pressure on nerves?	YES →	Less than a 50 percent chance of substantial relief of pain with surgery. Consider only if: 1. Appropriate nonsurgical therapy has been given an adequate chance to work. 2. Disability is substantial and not improving. 3. The same surgical procedure is recommended by at least two physicians, of whom at least one is a nonsurgical specialist in back problems.

NO ↓

An infrequent reason for back surgery (not discussed here) is being given. As a rule, the recommendation for surgery should come from at least two doctors, one of whom should not be a surgeon.

14
Heart Surgery

For almost 20 years after the first open-heart operation in 1952, heart surgery was concerned with the repair of damaged valves or congenital defects. The last 15 years have seen an explosion in surgery on the arteries that supply blood to the heart itself, coronary artery bypass grafting (CABG). The reason is straightforward: CABG is meant to relieve blockages caused by coronary artery disease (CAD), the number one cause of death in America and a disease so common that as many as 75 percent of American adults have it. Any therapy directed at coronary artery disease has the potential for being applied to millions of people—a gigantic potential for both benefit and harm. If it can help large portions of persons with CAD, then the greater the benefit. But if it cannot benefit a substantial portion, its use in these patients will be of great harm.

The concept of CABG is simple: A vein from another part of the body, usually the leg, is used to bypass a blocked portion of the coronary artery. It is attached to the artery above and below the obstruction. The operation itself is as delicate as the concept is simple. Placing the graft (the transplanted vein) on the artery of a living human heart so that blood

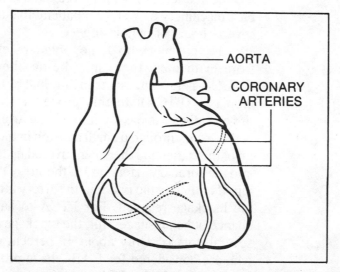

The coronary arteries supply the heart muscle with freshly oxygenated blood.

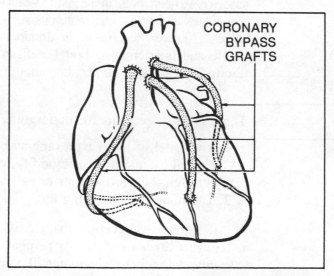

In coronary artery bypass surgery, a vein from another part of the body is used to bypass a blocked portion of a coronary artery. It is attached to the artery above and below the obstruction.

actually flows easily around the obstruction requires a dedicated team of health professionals using complex machinery as well as a patient able to undergo several hours of major surgery.

For patients who do not obtain relief of angina from medicines, there may be an alternative to CABG—percutaneous transluminal coronary angioplasty (PTCA). In this procedure, a balloon-tipped catheter is passed into a large artery, usually in the groin, through a small incision in the skin. The tip of the catheter is then maneuvered up to the heart into the coronary artery and to the site of the narrowing. By inflating the balloon, the artery is dilated and the blockage relieved. For PTCA to have a good chance of being successful, the blockage must meet several criteria. Only about 10 percent of patients who are considered for CABG have problems that can be treated with PTCA.

Surgery on valves and congenital defects is no less complex than CABG and may be more so. Real strides have been made in the last 15 years in improving techniques and prosthetic materials such as artificial valves. However, because of the dominant position of CABG and its potential for both benefit and harm, this discussion will focus on deciding about CABG.

Benefits

There are two reasons for undergoing CABG:

1. The relief of heart pain (angina pectoris) caused by insufficient blood flow through the coronary arteries
2. The hope of prolonging life.

It is generally accepted that CABG is effective in relieving angina—about 70 percent of patients have complete relief and another 20 percent experience partial relief. Some, perhaps most, of this relief comes from the intended effect of the surgery, i.e., to improve the blood flow to areas of the heart that have caused pain because of insufficient blood flow.

However, there are at least two ways in which the surgery could be credited with relieving pain even though it did not do so through the desired effect of improving blood flow. First, the heart tissue causing the pain may die (myocardial infarction) during the operation; dead tissue causes no pain. However, myocardial infarction is a heart attack, and may present its own set of serious problems even though pain is relieved. Second, it is known from previous studies of angina that a sham operation in which the chest is opened but nothing is done to the heart will bring relief in about 40 percent of patients. This is the placebo effect of surgery, and it is a very powerful one. Indeed, Dr. Bernandine Bulkley reviewed studies of patients undergoing CABG and found that the relief of pain was essentially the same in patients who had open grafts permitting blood flow and patients whose grafts had closed and were useless. This should temper your enthusiasm for CABG, but it is still a fact that there is a high probability of relief from angina through surgery if medical therapy (drugs, exercise programs, etc.) fails.

The effect of CABG on life expectancy is much less impressive. The best information suggests that life expectancy is improved only with certain kinds of problems of the coronary arteries. Specifically, benefits can be expected when there is almost complete obstruction of the most important artery, the left main coronary artery, or there is significant blockage of all three of the heart's principal arteries. In such patients, the increase in life expectancy with surgery as opposed to drugs has been estimated to be between six and 12 months.

Risks

As you would expect, the risk of surgery is related to the severity of the heart disease. Patients who have sustained considerable heart damage already have high risks and may not be candidates for surgery at all.

Risk is also related to the skill of the operating team, which is most easily measured by the number of procedures that it performs. It stands to reason that it is almost impossible for a team that only does one operation a week or a month to be as good as a team that averages one procedure a day.

Mortality rates have been reported to range between 1 percent and 20 percent. The very low percentage may be too optimistic since it suggests that surgery has been limited to essentially healthy people who may not have needed the operation the most. The very high percentage should not be seen in modern, responsible programs. The death rate for a competent surgical team operating on an "average" mix of patients should be 3 percent or 4 percent.

Five percent to 10 percent of patients will suffer a heart attack during surgery or immediately after. About 5 percent will suffer other serious complications such as excessive bleeding and serious infection. The mortality rate for patients undergoing PTCA is about 1 percent. About 7 percent of patients will have a complication such as prolonged angina, heart attack, or, rarely, rupture of the artery. The last usually requires that emergency CABG be performed. Prolonged angina may require elective CABG.

Costs

For people having coronary artery bypass grafting, a hospital stay of five to six days is optimal. The care given following this kind of surgery is very much like that given following a heart attack. The patient will spend one day in intensive care, staying overnight. He or she will then advance to a regular hospital room but continue to have careful monitoring. The average hospital stay for CABG surgery is 15 days. This average includes patients who had complications as well as those who were "routinely" admitted to the hospital for a specified number of days.

The average cost of CABG surgery is $21,800, but you can expect your bill to range between $13,000 and $31,000, depending on, among other factors, the region of the country in which the surgery is performed.

Making Decisions About Heart Surgery

There are three generally accepted criteria for considering CABG or PTCA:

1. Disabling angina persists despite optimal medical therapy.
2. The obstruction(s) is located where it can be approached surgically.
3. The heart is not already severely damaged.

Your doctors must decide on the last two factors, but you are the one who decides how severe the pain is. If the problem is one that can be treated with PTCA, it is the logical choice.

If pain is minor, but coronary arteriography (visualization of an artery by X-rays after injection of dye) has shown that survival would be improved with surgery, you have a difficult choice. Current statistics indicate that you may improve your life expectancy by having the operation, but most of the patients in these studies had substantial pain (that's why they were operated on). It is not clear that the results will be the same if you have little or no discomfort, since this may indicate less severe disease. There are also claims being made that newer drug therapies can improve the outcomes of patients not treated with surgery. In this situation it is best to obtain the recommendation of more than one physician, and at least one of your advisers should be an internist or cardiologist *not* associated with the cardiac surgery team.

The indications for surgery on defective valves and congenital defects are less controversial but depend on the specific kind of valve problem or congenital defect. The major question here is one of timing. It is rare for surgery to be done soon after discovering a defect. Most often it is necessary to do repeated studies over time to find out how severe the problem is and whether it is progressing. Although there is usually less difference of opinion about these kind of operations than about CABG, a second opinion can be useful in helping you to be certain that all alternatives have been adequately explored.

Heart Surgery

Is this CABG for the relief of angina?

→ YES → Surgery is appropriate if pain is substantial and medical (drug) therapy has failed. Opinion of second cardiologist, not a member of CABG team, is suggested. PTCA should be considered.

↓ NO

Is this CABG suggested as a means to prolong life?

→ YES → Increase in life expectancy demonstrated only when left main coronary artery or all three major coronary arteries have high degree of blockage. Second opinion suggested.

↓ NO

Is this surgery to repair a damaged valve or congenital defect?

→ YES → This could be any one of many different procedures. Indications for these procedures are less controversial than for CABG, but a second opinion may be helpful to you.

↓ NO

Surgery is being suggested for an unusual problem not discussed here. Second opinion may be helpful.

15
Cataracts

A cataract is a cloudiness that forms in the lens of the eye. Although cataracts may be present at birth (congenital cataracts) or occur as the result of an injury (traumatic cataract), most occur after the age of 60. Diabetics are more likely to form cataracts than nondiabetics. Most cataracts slowly become more and more dense until all vision is blocked. Currently, it is not possible to stop or reverse the progression of a cataract, and removal of the lens itself is the only way to restore vision.

Cataract surgery has changed remarkably in the last two decades. It used to be that the cataract had to become quite dense before it could be removed. And, following surgery, patients had to wear thick glasses that magnified objects by about 30 percent and greatly reduced peripheral vision. The technical problems of surgery and the less-than-satisfactory eyeglasses led to a standard but unhappy rule for cataract operations: You waited until you had virtually no vision before having the operation.

New technology has changed all this. New surgical techniques that use ultrasound (phacoemulsification) to liquify the lens or cold to freeze it (cryoex-

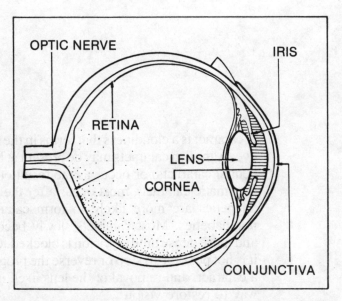

This illustration depicts the anatomy of the human eye. A cataract is a cloudiness that forms in the lens of the eye. Cataract surgery requires the removal of the lens.

traction) allow removal of the lens before the cataract becomes very dense.

Advances in the lenses used after the operation are equally important. Contact lenses magnify objects by only 5 percent to 10 percent and do not interfere with peripheral vision. However, handling the lenses may be a major problem for older patients, and this can be a barrier to their use in that age group. Fortunately, technology has provided an alternative to the contact lens in a tiny lens that is placed inside the eye (intraocular lens) at the time the natural lens is removed. An intraocular lens magnifies objects by only 1 percent to 3 percent and, of course, requires no handling by the patient. The disadvantage of the intraocular lens is that it requires a more difficult surgical procedure with increased risks of complications. Problems with intraocular lenses usually require another operation and the results may be poor. Clearly, it is easier to deal with a problem contact lens than a problem intraocular lens.

If you have a cataract in one eye, it is quite possible that you have at least the beginning of a cataract in the other eye. Nevertheless, it is unusual for cataract operations to be done on both eyes at the same time because of the increased risks of complications. Since these complications can lead to total loss of vision, most patients and surgeons are unwilling to run the risk of complete blindness in both eyes. Most often one cataract is more dense than the other and the rule is to remove this lens first. But there is a problem when only one eye is operated on: Although vision may be clearer in the eye from which the cataract has been removed, it will be different from that in the other eye simply because no artificial lens can exactly mimic a natural lens. Many individuals find this difference in vision difficult to tolerate. It is not unusual for patients to prefer using the eye not operated on, even though it may have a cataract and poorer vision, because things look more natural when viewed through that eye. The result is that most persons with cataracts in both eyes eventually consider surgery in the second eye even though they may have very good vision in one eye after the first operation.

Benefits

If there are no other problems with the eye that interfere with vision, successful removal of a cataract will restore good vision. In many cases vision will be almost perfect. Near-perfect results with respect to sharpness of vision ($20/20$ visual acuity) are somewhat more likely if contact lenses are chosen rather than intraocular lenses, since the contact lenses may be adjusted after the operation. However, intraocular lenses do not require the handling and care that contact lenses do.

Risks

Most cataract surgery does not require a stay in the hospital and can be done under local anaesthesia. Thus, the risk of death from a cataract operation is usually very low, probably less than one in 100,000.

The major risks of this surgery are complications that lead to loss of vision. Infections and bleeding into the eye are the greatest threats, although direct injury to the inside of the eye may also occur. The placement of an intraocular lens increases the risks somewhat and, of course, there may be problems with the lens itself.

Perhaps even more than in other types of surgery, the risk of complications depends on the skill of the surgeon. There are a number of different surgical techniques that may be used. You may hear these referred to as intracapsular, extracapsular, phacoemulsification, cryoextraction or some combination of these. Each has its advantages and disadvantages, and none is superior for all patients. But it is very important for your surgeon to have substantial experience in the procedure that is selected for you. When the surgeon has such experience, the risk of major complication is probably considerably less than one in 100. Without such experience, the same procedure may carry a risk of major complication as high as one in five or ten.

Costs

The optimal way for cataract surgery to be done is on an ambulatory basis. Still, the average hospital stay for cataract surgery is two days. This average includes cases in which there were complications and those in which the patient was "routinely" admitted for a couple of days.

You can expect the cost of cataract surgery to be about $2,400 for ambulatory surgery and between $3,000 and $5,000 for surgery and a hospital stay of two days. However, the cost of medical care varies considerably from one region of the country to another, and your final bill could be above or below this range.

Making Decisions About Cataract Surgery

If the cataract is not causing you any substantial difficulty, then surgery is of little benefit. You will want to wait until you know that the benefits of surgery will outweigh the risks and the other problems associated with the use of an artificial lens.

Damage to other parts of the eye may mean that vision will be little improved after cataract removal. This is most likely to occur if the retina has already been damaged by diabetes. Be sure that your physician determines that cataract removal will improve your vision substantially. New instruments are available to help in this determination.

Once you have determined that cataract removal will result in a substantial improvement in the quality of your life, be prepared for the hard work that follows the surgery. Vision will not be exactly the same in both eyes. If a contact lens is selected, you must develop the skills necessary for proper handling and care of the lens. If a cataract is present in the second eye, then surgery on that eye is likely to be a consideration.

For most patients, cataract surgery is safest when it is done on an ambulatory basis and under local anaesthesia. However, because of a quirk in the Medicare law, some surgeons are charging two or three times as much for an operation done on an ambulatory basis as they would for the same operation when the patient is admitted to the hospital. There is no justification for this. Unless there are specific medical reasons for admission to the hospital, you should have your surgery done on an ambulatory basis because this is the safest for you, *and* you should let your surgeon know that you expect the fee to be the same as it would be for an operation done in the hospital.*

* As this goes to press, it appears that the Medicare law will be changed to eliminate higher fees for ambulatory surgery.

Cataracts

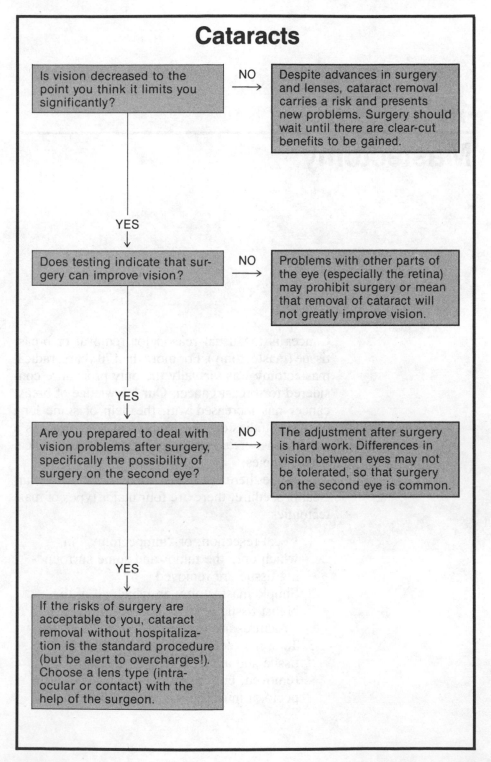

Is vision decreased to the point you think it limits you significantly?

→ NO → Despite advances in surgery and lenses, cataract removal carries a risk and presents new problems. Surgery should wait until there are clear-cut benefits to be gained.

YES ↓

Does testing indicate that surgery can improve vision?

→ NO → Problems with other parts of the eye (especially the retina) may prohibit surgery or mean that removal of cataract will not greatly improve vision.

YES ↓

Are you prepared to deal with vision problems after surgery, specifically the possibility of surgery on the second eye?

→ NO → The adjustment after surgery is hard work. Differences in vision between eyes may not be tolerated, so that surgery on the second eye is common.

YES ↓

If the risks of surgery are acceptable to you, cataract removal without hospitalization is the standard procedure (but be alert to overcharges!). Choose a lens type (intraocular or contact) with the help of the surgeon.

16
Mastectomy

Cancer is the usual reason for removal of breast tissue (mastectomy). For more than 70 years, radical mastectomy was virtually the only procedure considered for breast cancer. Our knowledge of breast cancer has increased with the help of some long overdue studies of the results of mastectomy. As a result, most breast operations today are not radical mastectomies.

While there are many minor variations in surgical procedure, there are four major types of mastectomies:

1. Local resection, or "lumpectomy," in which only the tumor and some surrounding tissue are removed
2. Simple mastectomy, in which all of the breast tissue is removed but no other structures are excised
3. Total mastectomy, in which all breast tissue and adjacent lymph nodes are removed, but the muscles of the chest (the pectoral muscles) are not disturbed

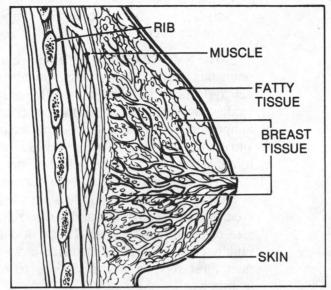

This illustration depicts the anatomy of the human breast.

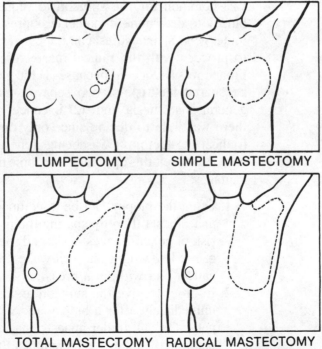

LUMPECTOMY   SIMPLE MASTECTOMY

TOTAL MASTECTOMY   RADICAL MASTECTOMY

The four major types of mastectomies result in incisions of varying size and shape.

4. Radical mastectomy in which breast tissue, pectoral muscles, and lymph nodes are removed.

The National Institutes of Health currently recommends total mastectomy for patients whose cancer appears to be confined to the breast. Some studies suggest that radiation therapy combined with lumpectomy is as good as total mastectomy in this situation, but most physicians advise total mastectomy. When cancer has spread beyond the breast, various combinations of mastectomy, radiation, and/or anticancer drugs (chemotherapy) will be considered, depending on extent and location of spread and size of the original tumor. This is a complex and rapidly changing area of medicine in which the patient must rely on her physicians to explain her alternatives.

Changes in procedures have brought changes in the way the procedures are chosen. In the past, it was common for the surgeon to request that the biopsy to determine if cancer was present be done under general anaesthesia and, if cancer was found, to proceed with the radical mastectomy. This approach was advocated because (1) the patient would be spared the risk of two separate exposures to general anaesthesia and, (2) if cancer was found, there was little to decide since only one operation (radical mastectomy) was being done for this disease. However, this approach has some major disadvantages:

1. Often the biopsy can be done under local anaesthesia thereby sparing the patient the risk of general anaesthesia and the anxiety of not knowing if she will wake up with cancer and without a breast.
2. In order to give the surgeon an answer immediately after a biopsy and while the patient is still under anaesthesia, the pathologist must use techniques that are less accurate than those that require hours or days to perform. Thus, the pressure for

an immediate answer means that errors in diagnosis are more likely to occur.

3. Participation by the patient in decision making is much more difficult, as she must deal with whether or not she has cancer and consider all treatment options in giving consent to the "all-in-one" procedure.

For these reasons, most patients and their physicians prefer to do a biopsy and then to discuss treatment options if cancer is found.

Benefits

Unfortunately, research has not been done that allows us to say exactly what the best approach to breast cancer is for every patient. Indeed, there has never been research to tell us how much benefit any treatment has over no treatment. We do know that the limited forms of surgery are as effective as radical mastectomy in most, if not all, patients for whom surgery is appropriate.

The addition of chemotherapy to mastectomy appears to be beneficial for premenopausal women in whom cancer is found in the lymph nodes under the arm. The benefit of adding it in other situations is less certain.

The prognosis for a patient with breast cancer depends far more on the amount of disease found during the operation than the surgical procedure used. For patients in whom there is no evidence that cancer has spread beyond the breast tissue itself, the chances of being tumor-free after five years and ten years are approximately 78 percent and 50 percent. For persons in whom cancer is found in the lymph nodes, the chances of being tumor-free at five and ten years are 50 percent and 33 percent. For those who have cancer spreading into the chest wall or skin, the five and ten year figures are 20 percent and 10 percent.

Risks

As you would expect, the risk of the simplest procedure is somewhat less than that for the more involved ones. But the difference is not that great, and in all cases, the risk of death appears to be less than one in 1,000.

The greatest difference is in the disability and disfigurement caused by a radical mastectomy. Swelling of the arm, which may be persistent, occurs in about 10 percent of radical mastectomies and less than 1 percent of the other procedures. Another 10 percent of those undergoing radical mastectomy will have weakness in their arm; this does not occur with the other procedures. The removal of the chest muscles in radical mastectomy makes breast reconstruction difficult or impossible and makes the use of an artificial breast (prosthesis) less satisfactory. Wound complications occur in about 15 percent of radical mastectomies and 5 percent to 10 percent of the other operations.

Costs

For a simple or total mastectomy, the optimal hospital stay is two days. For a radical mastectomy, it might be three days or more. Lumpectomies should be done on an ambulatory basis, as should breast biopsies. In addition, breast biopsies require only local anaesthesia. The average hospital stay for a mastectomy is eight days. This average includes patients who were "routinely" admitted to the hospital for a stay of several days.

The cost of a mastectomy will probably range between $2,200 and $8,000. However, the cost of medical care varies considerably from one region of the country to another, and your bill could wind up above or below this range.

Making Decisions About Mastectomy

As indicated above, we think it wise to separate biopsy from mastectomy so that diagnosis can be separated from therapy. If a diagnosis of cancer is made, the vast majority of women should not be facing radical mastectomy but should be considering the more limited procedures and the question of radiation therapy. As noted, research does not allow us to say what the best approach is at this time. The opinion of a medical oncologist, a non-surgical specialist in cancer, is most useful in helping you and your surgeon to choose an approach.

Mastectomy

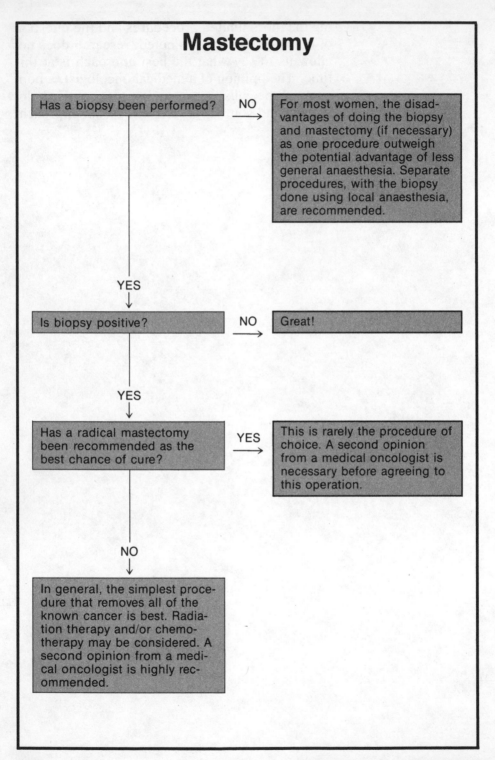

Has a biopsy been performed? → NO → For most women, the disadvantages of doing the biopsy and mastectomy (if necessary) as one procedure outweigh the potential advantage of less general anaesthesia. Separate procedures, with the biopsy done using local anaesthesia, are recommended.

YES

Is biopsy positive? → NO → Great!

YES

Has a radical mastectomy been recommended as the best chance of cure? → YES → This is rarely the procedure of choice. A second opinion from a medical oncologist is necessary before agreeing to this operation.

NO

In general, the simplest procedure that removes all of the known cancer is best. Radiation therapy and/or chemotherapy may be considered. A second opinion from a medical oncologist is highly recommended.

17
Knee Surgery

At one time, it appeared that there would be an operation to repair virtually all parts of the knee and that these operations would be performed frequently. Disappointment with the results of some of the procedures and the advent of arthroscopy (examination of the interior of a joint with a special instrument) have led to a decline in the number of standard surgical procedures on the knee.

The portions of the knee most often injured are the ligaments—tough, fibrous bands that hold the joint together—and the cartilage—discs of semi-rigid tissue that act as shock absorbers between the bones of the leg and the thigh.

Complete tears of the collateral ligaments (usually the medial collateral) are repaired by sewing the ends of the ligament together again; sometimes other tissues are moved to help strengthen this repair. A leg cast is then worn for six or seven weeks.

Cruciate ligaments are difficult to repair, and the results are often less than satisfactory. A number of procedures to repair cruciate ligaments have been used in the past but are performed infrequently now.

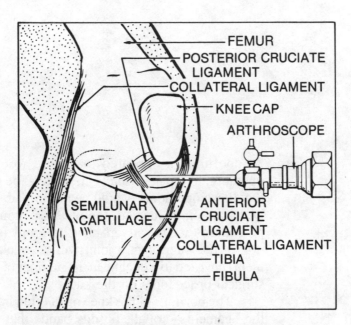

FEMUR
POSTERIOR CRUCIATE LIGAMENT
COLLATERAL LIGAMENT
KNEE CAP
ARTHROSCOPE
SEMILUNAR CARTILAGE
ANTERIOR CRUCIATE LIGAMENT
COLLATERAL LIGAMENT
TIBIA
FIBULA

In arthroscopy, a tube inserted into the knee joint allows the surgeon to see inside the joint. Using small instruments inserted through the arthroscope, the surgeon can remove torn cartilage.

Partial tears of ligaments (sprains) do not require surgery, but do benefit from rehabilitation through exercise.

Cartilage tears are probably more frequent than ligament damage. Torn cartilage is not repaired; it is simply removed. This may be accomplished through the use of an arthroscope, a small tube inserted into the knee joint that allows the surgeon to see the torn cartilage and often to remove it by using small instruments inserted through the arthroscope. The arthroscope causes less disability and requires less recovery time than a traditional operation in which the knee is cut open in order to expose the torn cartilage. Arthroscopic surgery usually does not require a stay in the hospital.

Benefits

Surgical repair of completely torn collateral ligaments decreases the risk of an unstable joint after recovery from the initial injury. This is especially important for athletes who cannot tolerate such instability. It may be less important for nonathletes who may choose to run the risk of an unstable knee in order to avoid the risk of surgery. It has been estimated that only about 25 percent of collateral ligament tears require surgery. When surgery is done, good to excellent results are obtained in about 75 percent of the cases. About 80 percent of patients who have cartilage removed will have good to excellent results immediately after their operation.

Risks

About 20 percent of those individuals who have surgery for torn collateral ligaments will continue to have some disability after the operation. About 5 percent will have some complication of the surgery, usually an infection of the skin or the joint itself. The most serious complication, pulmonary embolism, is a constant threat because of swelling of the knee and immobilization of the leg, both of which predispose to clot formation in the leg. The risk of death associated with this type of knee surgery is low, probably less than one in 5,000.

More than half of the persons who have surgery for torn cruciate ligaments continue to have some disability. Complications and risks are essentially the same as those experienced for collateral ligament repair.

Ten percent to 20 percent of persons who have cartilage removed may have some continuing problem immediately after surgery. However, there is some evidence that removal of cartilage increases the chance of arthritis in the knee years later; this may be a problem for another 10 percent to 20 percent of persons having the operation. When removal is done through an arthroscope, the risk of death is very low and is essentially the risk associated with the type of anaesthesia used. For general anaesthesia, this has been estimated at one in 10,000 to one in 100,000. For spinal or local anaesthesia, the risk is so low as to be impossible to estimate with any confidence.

Costs

Arthroscopy almost always should be an ambulatory procedure. For surgery in which the knee is opened (arthrotomy), a one-day hospital stay is optimal. Yet the average hospital stay for arthroscopy is three days, and for arthrotomy, it is four to five days. Of course, this average includes cases in which there were complications, but it also includes patients who were admitted to the hospital for longer stays than were necessary.

The cost of this surgery will be about $1,400 for arthroscopy done as ambulatory surgery. It should range between $2,000 and $4,000 for surgery and a hospital stay of four days. However, the cost of medical care varies considerably from one region of the country to another, and your bill could wind up above or below this range.

Making Decisions About Knee Surgery

The benefits of knee surgery are highly dependent on the individual. The professional or amateur athlete who believes continuing to compete is very important must consider surgery if he or she suffers a completely torn collateral ligament. If a cartilage problem makes life miserable, then it is time to consider removal. Arthroscopy is the choice here since it is less risky, more convenient, and less costly.

The best information available now indicates that surgery for torn cruciate ligaments is to be avoided in most cases.

A second opinion is useful here, especially when cartilage or cruciate ligaments are the problem. One study found that the second surgeon did *not* recommend surgery in about 40 percent of patients referred after a knee operation was suggested.

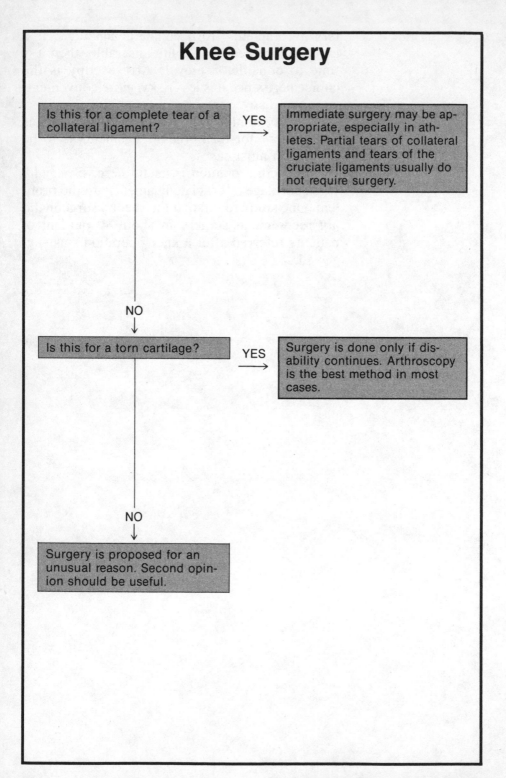

Knee Surgery

Is this for a complete tear of a collateral ligament?

YES → Immediate surgery may be appropriate, especially in athletes. Partial tears of collateral ligaments and tears of the cruciate ligaments usually do not require surgery.

NO ↓

Is this for a torn cartilage?

YES → Surgery is done only if disability continues. Arthroscopy is the best method in most cases.

NO ↓

Surgery is proposed for an unusual reason. Second opinion should be useful.

18
Hysterectomy

In discussions of unnecessary operations, hysterectomy is always a major topic. When it comes to operations done for a bad reason, a questionable reason, or no reason at all, it is rivaled only by a tonsillectomy and adenoidectomy (T&A). Hysterectomies have been done for everything from cancer to low back pain to depression. Surveys indicate that this operation is done at least twice as often in the United States as in Great Britain or western European countries. Studies carried out in Maine and Vermont showed that the rates at which hysterectomies are performed are three times higher in areas with the most gynecologists and surgeons. Altogether these studies strongly suggest that the most important factor in determining whether a hysterectomy is done is not the presence of any particular disease or condition, but the presence of a doctor who wants to do the operation.

The hysterectomy business is big business. It is the most frequently performed major operation in women. It has been estimated that the cost of a hysterectomy to a woman is well in excess of $10,000. This includes the cost of medical care, disability, work lost, tests, etc. Since medical care costs

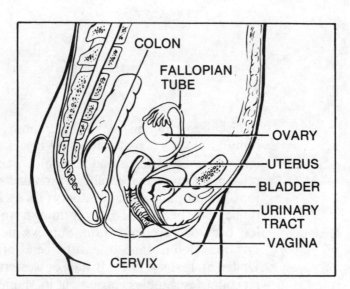

This illustration shows the location of the uterus in relation to other internal organs.

are almost always distributed to the rest of us through insurance mechanisms, each of us ends up helping to pay for many millions of dollars worth of hysterectomy surgery each year.

On the positive side, there are reasons for having a hysterectomy that are accepted by virtually everyone; these are listed in Table 18.1 on page 134. Each represents a disease in or near the uterus that is serious, may be life-threatening, and cannot be handled adequately without removal of the uterus.

On the negative side, there are reasons that are rarely, if ever, adequate for a hysterectomy and deserve our scorn. These include depression, low back pain not related to one of the conditions listed in Table 18.1, contraception only (there are safer methods available), and "because you don't need it anymore."

Hysterectomy decisions can be complicated by the fact that there are good reasons for the operation that are not clear cut but, rather, are subjective and depend on the woman's own feelings. A typical situation is a woman 40 to 50 years of age who has not undergone the menopause and is in good general health. However, she has substantial trouble with her menstrual periods. Perhaps she has heavy bleeding that has required a dilatation and curettage (D&C) on one or more occasions in the past. She may have painful periods as well. She complains of fatigue and may be slightly anemic, but the two probably are not related and she requires no therapy. Her Pap smears are normal, so cancer is not an indication for surgery. She wants no more children and would welcome a permanent form of contraception but fears major surgery.

Should this woman have a hysterectomy? As we shall see, the answer depends almost entirely on how the woman feels about the risks and benefits of this surgery.

Benefits

The most certain benefits in our example are relief of menstrual discomfort and inconvenience. Undoubtedly, the risk of cancer of the uterus will be removed. If the ovaries are removed as part of the procedure, the risk of cancer of the ovaries will also be removed. Unfortunately, removal of the ovaries will remove the source of female hormones and is likely to produce the symptoms associated with menopause—hot flashes, etc. However, this woman will not have to undergo any further D&Cs or use medicines for menstrual problems if she has the operation.

One study has concluded that there may be a slight (seven to 14 days) gain in life expectancy if an otherwise healthy 40-year-old woman has her uterus and ovaries removed. According to the estimates of this study, the gain is a result of the risk from cancer of the uterus and ovaries slightly exceeding the risk of death due to the operation or its complications. However, the authors of the study regard this as essentially a toss-up and point out that the presence of increased age or other medical problems would dramatically shift the risks the other way, i.e., the risks associated with the operation would far outweigh the risks associated with cancer in the future.

Risks

For a woman such as the one described above, the risk of death from hysterectomy is relatively small, probably less than one in 2,000. If the woman is older or has other medical problems, the risk could be much greater. For example, if the same woman had moderately severe hypertension, the risk of surgery presumably would be about ten times greater.

The most serious complication of hysterectomy is intestinal obstruction due to adhesions (fibrous scar tissue bands) in the abdomen. The incidence of such a complication might be as high as 1 percent in the ten years following the hysterectomy, and the mortality rate from the surgery necessary to relieve the obstruction (emergency laparotomy) has been estimated to be approximately 1 percent.

Less threatening but far more frequent complications include urinary tract infections, lingering discomfort, and disturbances in moods such as depression. Since these problems have not been well studied, little is known about their frequency and severity.

Costs

The optimal hospital stay for a vaginal hysterectomy is three days; for an abdominal hysterectomy, it is four. The average length of stay for a hysterectomy, though, is seven days. This average includes cases in which there were complications as well as patients who were "routinely" admitted to the hospital for several days.

The cost of a hysterectomy will probably range between $2,500 and $6,000, depending on the length of stay. However, the cost of medical care varies considerably from one region of the country to another, and your final bill could be above or below this range.

Making Decisions About Hysterectomy

Except when one of the first four conditions in Table 18.1 is present, the critical factor in making a decision about having a hysterectomy is your feelings about your symptoms and the risks of surgery. Even if age or other medical problems actually tilt the risk equation slightly against surgery, it still may be worth the risk if symptoms are severe and disabling. The essential point is that only you can decide how much relieving the symptoms is worth and only you can decide how to value the risk of surgery *now* versus the risk of cancer *later*. For most women, neither the risk of surgery nor the risk of cancer is so large as to preclude consideration of both choices.

If a hysterectomy is decided upon, then the question of whether or not the ovaries will be removed must be considered. If menopause has occurred, the choice would seem to be straightforward: Removal adds little to the risk of surgery, it removes the risk of cancer of the ovaries, and it cannot have an effect on any postmenopausal symptoms. If menopause has not occurred, then you must weigh the immediate occurrence of the symptoms associated with menopause against the slight risk of cancer of the ovaries. An obvious compromise, removing one of the ovaries and leaving one, is not uncommon and does prevent the immediate occurrence of symptoms associated with menopause. However, there is no research available to specify exactly its impact on the risk of cancer.

For most women, time will help clarify the situation. There is no need to rush into surgery at the first sign of a menstrual problem, nor is it necessary to forever avoid surgery if symptoms continually cause discomfort and disability.

Table 18.1   Indications for Hysterectomy

1. Cancers of the vagina, cervix, uterus, ovaries, or Fallopian tubes
2. Noncancerous diseases of the Fallopian tubes and ovaries where the uterus should be removed because of its closeness and involvement in the disease, e.g., chronic advanced tubal infection, extensive endometriosis
3. Involvement of the uterus in disease originating elsewhere, e.g., uterine involvement in colon cancer or in an abscess secondary to diverticulitis
4. Major complications of childbirth, e.g., uncontrollable bleeding, uterine rupture, uncontrolled uterine infection, etc.
5. Noncancerous diseases of the uterus causing severe symptoms, such as uterine pain or bleeding not responsive to hormonal therapy or uterine pain or bleeding in women in whom hormonal therapy is contraindicated
6. Late complications of childbirth including conditions related to supporting structures, e.g., cystocele, rectocele, procidentia.

Hysterectomy

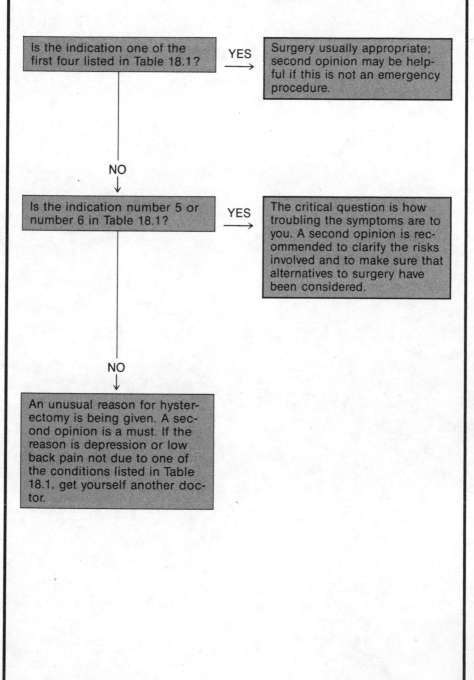

Is the indication one of the first four listed in Table 18.1?

YES → Surgery usually appropriate; second opinion may be helpful if this is not an emergency procedure.

NO ↓

Is the indication number 5 or number 6 in Table 18.1?

YES → The critical question is how troubling the symptoms are to you. A second opinion is recommended to clarify the risks involved and to make sure that alternatives to surgery have been considered.

NO ↓

An unusual reason for hysterectomy is being given. A second opinion is a must. If the reason is depression or low back pain not due to one of the conditions listed in Table 18.1, get yourself another doctor.

Part V

MEDICAL ADMISSIONS

Medical admissions are usually more complex than those for elective surgery. People having surgery know what is wrong with them and what is going to be done. But what about someone with chest pain or gastrointestinal bleeding? Problems like these cannot be treated until their causes are determined. Therefore, patients admitted to the hospital for medical reasons are likely to undergo a variety of tests.

If you require treatment for a medical problem, it is important to determine if hospitalization is actually necessary. Admission to the hospital is appropriate if you require complex therapy that cannot be administered any other way, if your condition requires close, round-the-clock monitoring, or if you need complex diagnostic tests that cannot be done on an outpatient basis. Hospitalization is appropriate when complications of a chronic disease or its therapy pose a serious threat.

The chapters in this part of the book discuss the primary reasons for medical admissions to the hospital. Of course, there are others. For all medical conditions, it is important to look into all of your options. The costs, benefits, and risks of hospitalization have to be evaluated. Remember that you have a one-in-five chance of suffering some kind of mishap or disability while you are in the hospital.

As a rule, hospitalization should be reserved for extremely serious medical problems. Beware of admissions for tests or a "workup." And never go for a rest.

19

Chest Pain and Heart Attack

Chest pain that suggests the possibility of a heart attack (myocardial infarction) is one of the most frequent reasons for admission to the hospital. However, less than half of the patients admitted will be found actually to have had a myocardial infarction; heart pain (angina pectoris) without myocardial infarction is the reason for chest pain in many of the remaining patients. While blockage (occlusion) in a coronary artery is the usual cause of both myocardial infarction and angina, the blockage is so severe in a myocardial infarction that there is death of heart tissue (an infarct). In angina there is no death of tissue.

Other problems that are not related to the heart at all, such as esophageal spasm, can mimic heart pain. Unfortunately, there are no tests that will quickly distinguish between heart attacks and other problems. For example, in the earliest stages of the heart attack, the electrocardiogram (heart tracing) may show either little or no change or changes that do not distinguish between a myocardial infarction and angina.

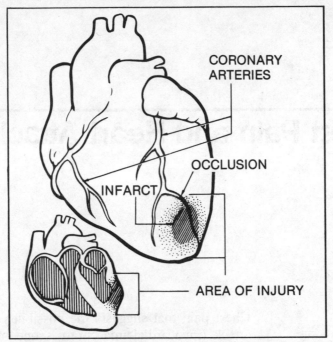

CORONARY
ARTERIES

OCCLUSION

INFARCT

AREA OF INJURY

Pain in the center of the chest is the main symptom of angina. This pain can spread to the throat, jaw, arms and back.

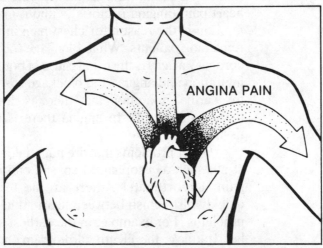

ANGINA PAIN

In the most common type of heart attack, a blockage in one of the coronary arteries cuts off the blood supply to one region of the heart muscle. The inadequate blood supply damages the tissue in that region.

The physician's task is to determine whether there is a *reasonable possibility* of a heart attack. However, it is difficult and dangerous to attempt to distinguish between angina and myocardial infarction. In practice, then, this means determining whether or not there is a reasonable chance that this is heart pain. Except for some elderly patients, it is generally agreed that the hospital is the place for persons experiencing myocardial infarction. Since an immediate diagnosis of myocardial infarction is usually not possible, the physician must admit many patients who will ultimately prove not to have had a myocardial infarction in order not to miss those who do.

Whether or not a myocardial infarction has occurred can usually be determined within the first 24 hours of hospitalization through the use of electro-cardiograms and blood tests. The medical jargon for this type of admission is "rule out MI," indicating that the diagnosis of myocardial infarction is not certain.

Patients known to have had a myocardial infarction and rule-out-MI patients will be admitted to the coronary care unit (CCU) if such a unit is available. CCUs specialize in intensive monitoring of the patient's heart function and vital signs and are equipped to respond immediately to complications, especially abnormalities of the heartbeat. Patients who are confirmed to have had a myocardial infarction but who have no complications (persistent abnormal rhythms, heart failure) usually remain in the CCU for two or three days; this is when complications are most likely to occur. They are then transferred to a regular hospital room or, in some hospitals, another specialty area where the monitoring of heart rhythm is continued; the other types of monitoring and observation are much less intense though, and life is somewhat closer to normal for the patient.

The total hospital stay for an uncomplicated myocardial infarction should be five to seven days. In the past, it was not unusual for MI patients to be kept at strict bed rest for three weeks or more. As the hazards of bed rest and hospitalization have become more appreciated, the period of hospitalization has been progressively shortened. Some physicians believe that a patient with an uncomplicated MI should be discharged after five days of hospitalization.

Patients who are found not to have had a myocardial infarction should be out of the CCU within 24 hours in almost all instances. If the diagnosis is clear and presents no threat (e.g., esophageal spasm), the patient can be discharged from the hospital even though it makes some physicians uncomfortable to discharge a patient directly from the CCU. If the diagnosis is not clear and further testing will be required, it has been common in the past to keep the patient in the hospital until the diagnostic tests can be completed. However, because of the risks and costs of continued hospitalization, many physicians will discharge the patient and continue the testing outside of the hospital if the patient does not require the monitoring or treatment capabilities of the hospital.

Angina patients often present the most difficult decisions in this regard. A severe episode of angina does not have the same potential for causing immediate problems as a heart attack. However, studies show that over the long term (six months and beyond), their prognosis is not very different from that of patients who have had myocardial infarction. Thus, the angina patient is not likely to benefit from being put in the coronary care unit or the hospital but does need special attention over the long term. This special attention may include further diagnostic testing. It may be reasonable to do some portion of this testing in the hospital as a part of rule-out-MI admission, but it is important to understand that the primary need is for an effective treatment *outside* the hospital.

Benefits

It is generally accepted that CCUs reduce the death rate in myocardial infarction, but how much it is reduced has been controversial. The most frequent estimates show that the CCU can reduce the death rate by between 5 percent and 10 percent. The benefit of being admitted to a hospital without a CCU is likely to be lower, although there is little research available on this question.

Several British studies have suggested that elderly patients (over age 70) with uncomplicated myocardial infarctions are an exception. These studies found that such patients actually had lower death rates when they were allowed to go home rather than when they were admitted to the CCU or hospital. American physicians are still reluctant to send any patient with a myocardial infarction home, perhaps because they believe that the patient and the patient's family expect hospitalization and/or they fear malpractice suits.

Risks

The continuous monitoring and activity of the CCU create a very abnormal and stressful environment for patients despite the best attempt of doctors and nurses to make it otherwise. The use of powerful drugs and procedures doesn't help either. As indicated above, this risk appears to outweigh the benefits in patients with acute myocardial infarction with the exception of the elderly.

For patients who do not have myocardial infarction, the CCU must be assumed to present at least the risk of a random medical admission and probably more. As indicated in Chapter 1, some studies suggest that the risk of death for such admissions could be as high as 1 percent. The major risks are due to drug reactions, infections, and pulmonary emboli.

Costs

A 24-hour hospital stay is optimal for individuals complaining of chest pain who are determined not to have suffered heart attacks: It takes that long to "rule out MI." Those who have had a myocardial infarction optimally should stay in the hospital five to seven days. The average length of stay for people with angina is three days; for those who have had heart attacks it is ten days. These averages include hospital stays that were longer than optimal because of complication or because the patient was "routinely" admitted to the hospital for several days.

Someone with chest pain that is not a heart attack can expect a hospital bill ranging between $1,000 and $2,000. Those who have had a heart attack probably will pay between $3,000 and $7,000. It is important to remember that the cost of medical care varies considerably from one region of the country to another, and your bill could wind up above or below this range.

Making Decisions About Hospitalization for Chest Pain

Unless the electrocardiogram shows the clear and unmistakable signs of a new myocardial infarction (and this is usually not the case), the decision to enter the hospital should be a judgment based on symptoms and physical examination. Rendering a professional opinion is the physician's responsibility, but you must understand the uncertainty of the situation and the risks involved in the admission decision. Most physicians believe that patients think hospitalization is good care and that they do not understand the risks of hospitalization. Let the doctor know that you understand the risks, and make the decision to enter the hospital by weighing the benefits against the risks.

If you are admitted to the hospital, your goal is to obtain the benefits of the hospital—a capacity for monitoring and quick treatment—while minimizing your exposure to the risks. If myocardial infarction is ruled out, you should seek discharge as soon as possible, as mentioned above, keeping in mind that on some occasions continued hospitalization will be appropriate.

If myocardial infarction is confirmed but there are no complications, early transfer from the CCU and early discharge from the hospital are desirable in most cases. Some physicians prefer to keep the patient in the hospital for longer periods specifically for the purpose of administering an exercise stress test ten days to two weeks after the myocardial infarction. Although such tests may be useful in prognosis, we think that a prolonged hospitalization for this purpose is unwise because it increases the risks to the patient, and the information gained is seldom useful in making decisions about therapy. If the physician feels strongly that a stress test is useful, it can be done later on an ambulatory basis with less risk to the patient.

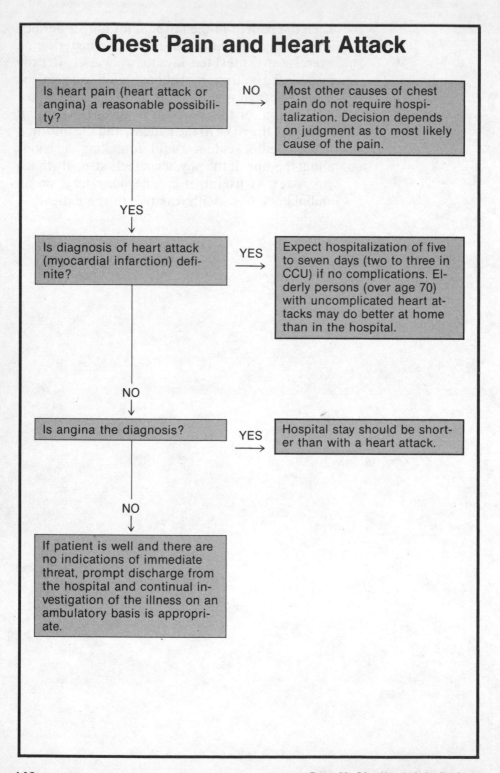

Chest Pain and Heart Attack

Is heart pain (heart attack or angina) a reasonable possibility?

NO →

Most other causes of chest pain do not require hospitalization. Decision depends on judgment as to most likely cause of the pain.

YES ↓

Is diagnosis of heart attack (myocardial infarction) definite?

YES →

Expect hospitalization of five to seven days (two to three in CCU) if no complications. Elderly persons (over age 70) with uncomplicated heart attacks may do better at home than in the hospital.

NO ↓

Is angina the diagnosis?

YES →

Hospital stay should be shorter than with a heart attack.

NO ↓

If patient is well and there are no indications of immediate threat, prompt discharge from the hospital and continual investigation of the illness on an ambulatory basis is appropriate.

20
Abdominal Pain and Gastrointestinal Bleeding

When the cause of acute abdominal pain or active gastrointestinal bleeding is not known, patients usually are admitted to the medical service, even though there is a strong possibility of surgery. Surgeons and physicians agree that making a rigorous attempt to arrive at a specific diagnosis is the most important thing to do in this situation. But since the surgeon is more interested in operating and diagnosis is the province of the internist, usually you will be admitted to a medical service under the care of an internist (or family physician) if the cause of the problem is unknown.

However, the need for a diagnosis alone is not a sufficient reason for being admitted to the hospital. Virtually all the tests that are used to diagnose abdominal pain or gastrointestinal bleeding can be done on an ambulatory basis. The need must be for diagnosis *without delay*. This "need for speed" often relates to the fact that a delay in surgery for some conditions increases the risk to the patient. However, it is also true that surgery greatly increases the risk to the patient if the problem turns out to be one that does not require it.

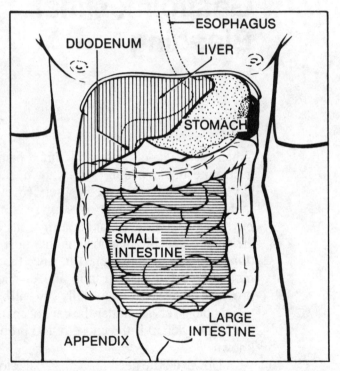

This illustration depicts the major organs within the abdomen.

Other reasons for hospitalization are the ability to monitor the patient's condition closely, to provide intravenous fluids, and to control carefully the types and amounts of medication. If the problem is active bleeding from the upper gastrointestinal tract (esophagus, stomach, or duodenum), vigorous attempts to control the bleeding without surgery will be made. Even if surgery will eventually be necessary for the problem, every attempt will be made to stabilize the situation by stopping or slowing the bleeding and replacing lost blood and fluids.

Benefits

Providing surgery without undue delay for those conditions for which it is indicated (appendicitis, ectopic pregnancy, etc.) is the principal objective of hospitalization. The hospital offers quick access to consultation with other physicians and to diagnostic tests.

It also offers careful management of medical therapy with intravenous fluids and medicines; often the greatest threat to the patient is not the disease that caused the problem, but rather the acute loss of blood or body fluids (dehydration). If this loss is controlled, the situation may become much less threatening and may not require more risky approaches such as surgery.

Risks

As a patient, you will use many of the resources of the hospital—monitoring, testing, therapy—and will be exposed to their inherent risks. The risk of surgery, if it is required, may be added to this. Since there is a wide range of tests and treatments for persons with abdominal pain or gastrointestinal bleeding, there is also a wide range of risks. The range for mortality rates is probably from 1 in 10,000 for the least sick patient to 1 in 5 for the severely ill.

Costs

In determining the optimal length of stay for people admitted to the hospital with abdominal pain, a basic rule applies: Unless the doctor finds something that requires hospital treatment, the patient should go home in two days or less. A diagnosis should be made as quickly as possible, usually within 24 hours, never more than 48 hours.

For those cases in which a specific problem is diagnosed, the optimal length of stay varies. For example, people requiring immediate surgery for acute appendicitis or cholecystitis should optimally stay one or two days. Those suffering from bleeding in the upper G.I. tract may go home 24 hours after the bleeding stops. People with pancreatitis or intestinal obstruction must stay until the problem is resolved.

The average length of stay for all people admitted to the hospital with abdominal pain is three days. For those with ulcers, it is seven days. These averages include patients who had complications as well as those who were "routinely" admitted to the hospital for several days.

If you are admitted to the hospital because of abdominal pain, you can expect your hospital bill to range between $2,000 and $5,000. Of course, the longer you stay in the hospital, the higher your bill will be. Keep in mind, though, that the cost of medical care varies considerably from one region of the country to another, and your final bill could be above or below this average.

| **Making Decisions About Hospitalization for Abdominal Pain and Gastrointestinal Bleeding** | The benefits outweigh the risks of hospitalization when you are in a situation that requires a quick diagnosis and the resources of the hospital while the diagnosis is being made. With respect to abdominal pain, this usually means that the pain is acute and is the type of pain that may be associated with one of the problems requiring surgery. Chronic pain can be investigated on an ambulatory basis and should rarely be the reason for admission to the hospital. Nausea and vomiting often accompany acute abdominal pain and may produce dehydration. If this dehydration cannot be treated |

adequately on an ambulatory basis, hospitalization may be needed.

Vomiting bright red blood or passing black tarry stools indicates substantial and active bleeding; admission to the hospital is required. Vomiting material that looks like coffee grounds is indicative of bleeding in the recent past; this is usually reason for admission unless there is reasonable assurance that bleeding is not active and the hematocrit (blood count) is normal.

Passage of large amounts of red blood through the rectum is unusual; hospitalization is the rule when it does occur. Small amounts of bright red blood on the stool or toilet paper most often are due to hemorrhoids or fissures; investigation of this problem should not require hospitalization. A positive test for hidden blood in the stool (Hemoccult, Detecatest, etc.) is not cause for hospitalization unless there is a severe anemia also. When severe anemia is present, the patient has little reserve, so an episode of active bleeding might pose a much greater risk than a person with a normal blood count. The physician may recommend hospitalization as a precaution against this combination of circumstances.

Abdominal Pain and Gastrointestinal Bleeding

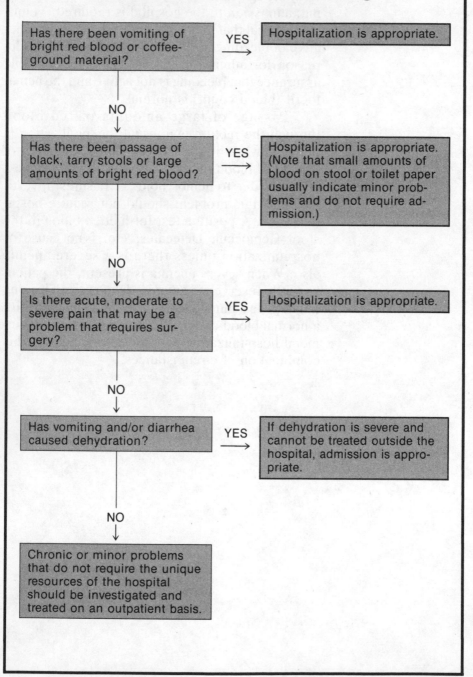

Has there been vomiting of bright red blood or coffee-ground material?

YES → Hospitalization is appropriate.

NO ↓

Has there been passage of black, tarry stools or large amounts of bright red blood?

YES → Hospitalization is appropriate. (Note that small amounts of blood on stool or toilet paper usually indicate minor problems and do not require admission.)

NO ↓

Is there acute, moderate to severe pain that may be a problem that requires surgery?

YES → Hospitalization is appropriate.

NO ↓

Has vomiting and/or diarrhea caused dehydration?

YES → If dehydration is severe and cannot be treated outside the hospital, admission is appropriate.

NO ↓

Chronic or minor problems that do not require the unique resources of the hospital should be investigated and treated on an outpatient basis.

21

Low Back Pain

Odds are that you will have low back pain some time during your life—more than 70 percent of us do. Fifty percent of those who experience back pain will go on to have three or more recurrences. The sad fact is that more than one-third of us will have multiple episodes of back pain spread over a number of years.

The good news is that more than 90 percent of these back pain episodes are completely resolved within two months regardless of what sort of treatment is instituted. The number of episodes does not influence the severity or duration of future recurrences. Most people with recurring back pain will have many minor episodes rather than a progressive increase in the severity of the problem.

The hospital offers little when it comes to low back pain. Virtually all specialists in this area regard exercise and protective body mechanics—learning how to lift, sit, etc.—as the keys to managing low back pain over the long term. Treatment for back pain, when it first begins, does not require the hospital and has become standardized: 24 to 78 hours of bed rest, pain relievers, and muscle relaxants. The use of traction to relieve pressure on the spine is now

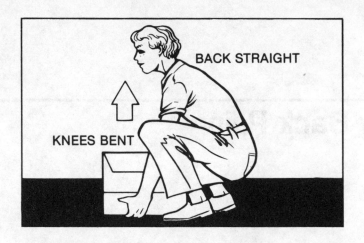

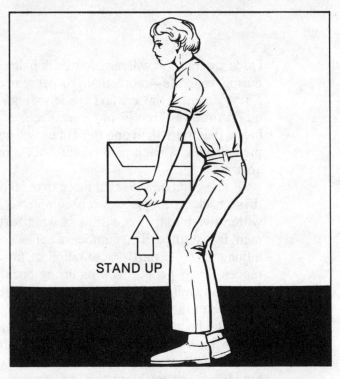

Lifting properly is good preventive medicine for back pain. It is important to bend your knees and keep your back straight when lifting. Also, don't try to lift anything that you think might be too heavy.

regarded as ineffective; it's only benefit being that it requires lying flat on your back in bed.

X-rays are always done and seldom helpful. The common abnormalities of the spine (disc space narrowing, bone spurs, joint asymmetry, spondylolisthesis, etc.) are found so frequently in people with and without back pain that they are of little use in determining treatment and predicting outcome. Almost everyone over the age of 50 will be found to have one of these X-ray abnormalities regardless of whether they have ever had any back pain. Perhaps the most beneficial use of X-rays is to detect unequal leg lengths in young people; the use of simple shoe inserts often takes care of the problem forever. Special X-rays (lumbar myelogram or CT scan) will be required should surgery ever be considered. In any event, all of these X-rays can be done without admission to the hospital.

The hospital should be used only by those in whom continued pressure on the nerves in the back threatens to cause permanent problems. In other words, it should be used only when surgery is being actively considered. As discussed in Chapter 13, this is usually indicated by weakness in the leg (foot drop).

Pain running down the leg into the foot (sciatica) is not a reliable indicator of a severe problem. In fact, sciatica is treated the same as low back pain without sciatica unless it is persistent and severe.

Benefits

The primary benefit to entering the medical service of a hospital for low back pain is that it may keep you off the surgical service. Bed rest, optimal use of medicines for pain relief and muscle relaxation, and frequent observations may lead to the conclusion that the problem is actually getting better rather than worse. This determination must be made as quickly as possible, usually within 24 to 48 hours.

Risks

Unfortunately, hospitalization for low back pain can provide the most dramatic illustrations of the hidden hazards of hospitalization. The bed rest meant to put back muscles at ease and relieve spasm is inactivity of the most serious sort. The other inherent risks of hospitalization—infection, mistakes, inherent risks of drugs and procedures—are present as well, of course. Since most persons with low back pain are otherwise quite healthy, a severe problem due to hospitalization seems all the more unexpected and tragic. No precise figures are available, but it seems prudent to assume that the mortality risk may approach that of unselected admissions to the medical service, estimated to be as high as 1 percent.

Costs

The average hospital stay for treatment of back pain is seven days, despite the fact that the hospital is seldom the best place for treatment.

The cost of hospitalization for low back pain will probably range between $2,000 and $5,000. However, the cost of medical care varies considerably from one region of the country to another, and your final bill could be above or below this range.

Making Decisions About Hospitalization for Low Back Pain

Evidence of nerve compression resulting in leg weakness is the primary reason to consider hospitalization for low back pain.

Your chances to consider carefully the alternatives to surgery for nerve compression may be increased by being admitted to the medical service rather than directly to the surgical service. Note that severity of back pain itself is not a prime consideration. Muscle spasm is usually the cause of this pain and the therapy for it (bed rest, pain reliever, muscle relaxant) is available to you at home. Occasionally, there may be sciatica involved, and the question of leg weakness may be difficult to resolve. In such a situation, hospitalization may be appropriate. If you are hospitalized, it is critical that a decision to return home or to perform surgery be made as quickly as possible. Otherwise, the risk of continued inactivity and exposure to the hospital environment will outweigh the benefits.

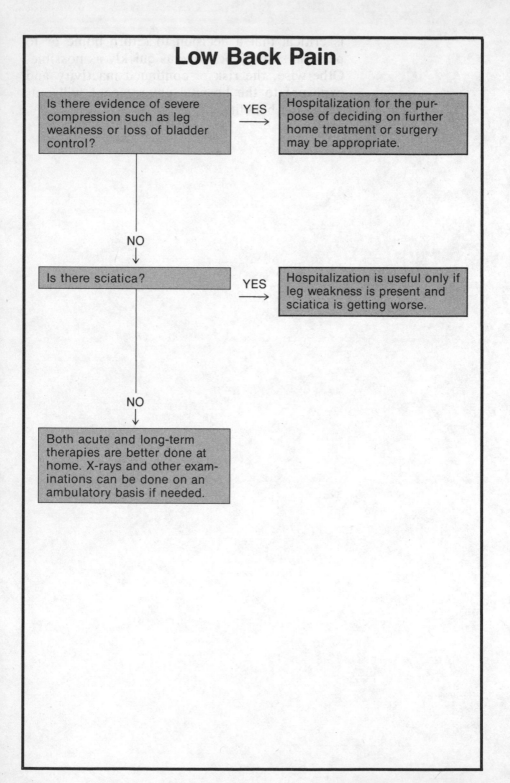

Low Back Pain

Is there evidence of severe compression such as leg weakness or loss of bladder control?

YES →

Hospitalization for the purpose of deciding on further home treatment or surgery may be appropriate.

NO ↓

Is there sciatica?

YES →

Hospitalization is useful only if leg weakness is present and sciatica is getting worse.

NO ↓

Both acute and long-term therapies are better done at home. X-rays and other examinations can be done on an ambulatory basis if needed.

22
Chronic Diseases

Congestive heart failure, emphysema, arthritis, kidney failure and diabetes are all examples of chronic diseases. There are others, of course.

By definition, chronic diseases cannot be cured. The goal of treatment is to minimize their impact so that life can proceed as normally as possible. If you have a chronic disease, the key to a vigorous and productive life is not what the medical system can do for you but what you can do for yourself with the help of your physician. Chronic diseases usually require some daily treatment as well as continual monitoring of signs and symptoms. If you are to be independent and active, you should take responsibility for your own treatment and monitoring. Competent physicians recognize that their most important responsibility is to teach you how to care for yourself.

The use of the hospital in chronic diseases usually represents a failure in management of the disease. Such failures do not necessarily indicate that you or your physician made an error, but they do mean that the primary goal of treatment has not been achieved. While hospitalization is disappointing for both patient and physician, it is important to recognize that use of the hospital is appropriate when complications of the disease or its therapy pose a serious threat to the patient. This happens to the best patients and the best doctors. The key, as always, is to make sure that the situation requires the special resources of the hospital.

Unfortunately, hospitalization may be suggested for other reasons. These hospitalizations often are not justified, usually because they do not help the patient to manage the chronic disease in everyday life.

For example, some physicians have routinely admitted newly diagnosed diabetic patients to the hospital for "workup and initial stabilization." At first glance, this seems to make some sense. Why not use the hospital to do all the tests that are necessary and make sure that the dosage of insulin and/or other medicines is just right? After all, managing diabetes will be a lifelong task for the patient, and it seems worthwhile to get it right from the beginning. The problem is that the primary goal is not to demonstrate that doctors and nurses can control the diabetes in the hospital, but rather to demonstrate that the patient can manage the disease as a part of his or her everyday activities. This is especially true in diabetes, since insulin requirements usually decline in the first few months of therapy. More importantly, insulin requirements ultimately depend on activity and diet, so it is important for the dosage to be tailored to the patient's everyday activities and diet rather than to the artificial circumstances imposed by hospitalization. Finally, the tests used in diabetes are available outside the hospital. Hospitalization may be needed when diabetes is first diagnosed because of complications, but it is not necessary simply because diabetes has just been diagnosed.

Similar admissions may be proposed for other chronic diseases such as heart disease or emphysema. Usually, the situation is the same: The goal is for stabilization in everyday life, not in the artificial environment of the hospital, and the tests needed are available without the patient being hospitalized. The hospital's brand of stabilization should be saved for those situations that pose a serious threat to the patient, in which the need is for stabilization without delay.

A similar reason for hospitalization is for a "tune-up." If monitoring or treatment of the disease is not going well, it is tempting to think that a stay in the hospital is a good way to get back on track. The problem here is the same: Getting it together in the hospital is not the goal. Managing the disease outside the hospital in everyday life is what counts.

There may come a time when the patient can no longer care for himself or herself despite the best efforts of all concerned. It is important to determine whether this means that the patient needs hospital care, skilled nursing care, or assistance in the activities of daily life. Most often it is one of the latter two situations, and the most appropriate response is assistance at home, home health care, or a nursing home. The hospital should not be seen as a source of nursing care only. The risk is too great, and the cost is too high.

Finally, a suggestion of hospitalization for the purpose of getting a rest should be rejected. As discussed in Part I, the hospital is no place to get a rest. It makes no sense to risk your health and your life and spend your money to find this out.

Benefits

When the threat to the patient is serious and treatment is needed immediately, hospitalization can turn around a quickly deteriorating situation and put the patient back on the road to successful management of the disease. It is no exaggeration to say that appropriate hospitalization may save lives, prevent disability, or restore some measure of lost function.

Risks

The patient admitted with chronic disease will have full exposure to the inherent risks of hospitalization. The use of multiple tests and multiple drugs can be assumed. The chronic disease itself may make the patient more susceptible to infections. There is a tendency to become much less active in the hospital, to try to get a rest, and this inactivity increases the hazards. Because of these risks and the problems posed by the chronic disease itself, the risk of death may even exceed the one in 100 chance reported in studies of medical admissions to the hospital.

Costs

Hospital stays for chronic diseases vary greatly in length. If the patient responds quickly to therapy, the stay will be very short. Sometimes, though, because of the ongoing nature of the disease, the stay can be prolonged. The average hospital stay for chronic disease is about seven days. This average includes hospital stays that were longer than optimal because of complications or failure to find more appropriate therapy.

The cost of hospitalization for a chronic disease will probably range between $1,500 and $7,000. The size of the bill is largely determined by the length of stay. However, the cost of medical care varies from one region of the country to another, and your final bill could be above or below this average.

Making Decisions About Hospitalization and Chronic Diseases

Taking the risk of hospitalization does not seem justified solely for the purpose of obtaining diagnostic tests or making adjustments in therapy. The only exception to this would be when the condition of the patient is deteriorating rapidly and a quick response is required. The hospital is simply not the place for a tune-up or rest. It is a risky and expensive way to obtain nursing care or housekeeping services. These concerns are summarized by the way that most physicians look at hospitalization for themselves and their families: Don't go unless you're really sick.

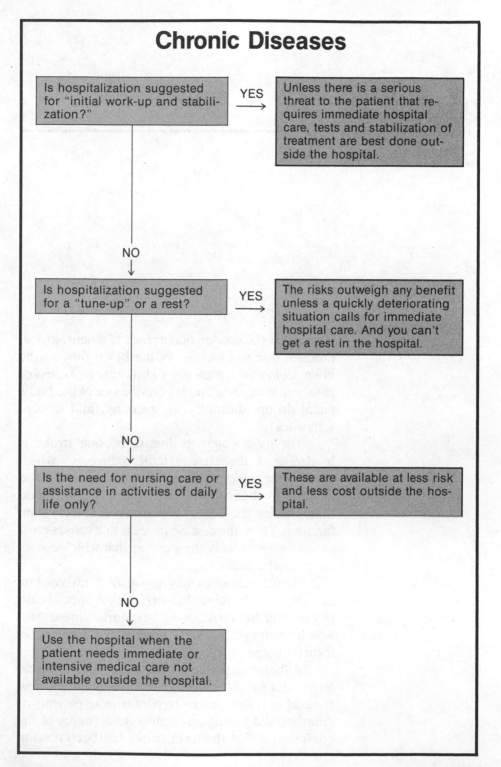

Chronic Diseases

Is hospitalization suggested for "initial work-up and stabilization?"

YES → Unless there is a serious threat to the patient that requires immediate hospital care, tests and stabilization of treatment are best done outside the hospital.

NO ↓

Is hospitalization suggested for a "tune-up" or a rest?

YES → The risks outweigh any benefit unless a quickly deteriorating situation calls for immediate hospital care. And you can't get a rest in the hospital.

NO ↓

Is the need for nursing care or assistance in activities of daily life only?

YES → These are available at less risk and less cost outside the hospital.

NO ↓

Use the hospital when the patient needs immediate or intensive medical care not available outside the hospital.

23
Stroke

A stroke is the sudden occurrence of a neurological problem due to blockage of the blood flow to the brain. Common symptoms of stroke are weakness or paralysis in the arm and leg on one side of the body, facial droop, difficulty in speaking, and unconsciousness.

The most common disease causing stroke is hardening of the arteries (atherosclerosis), which narrows the arteries that supply the brain with blood and causes clots to form. The clots block the blood flow, causing the death of brain tissue (cerebral infarction). Thus, the disease process that causes most strokes is essentially the same as that which causes most heart attacks.

However, strokes may also result from bleeding into the brain (cerebral hemorrhage). A special case of cerebral hemorrhage is a ruptured aneurysm, which occurs when a weak point in a cerebral vessel forms a bulge (aneurysm) and then bursts.

Although a stroke is one of the oldest medical terms and has been recognized for centuries, few medical problems are more confusing to patients or controversial among physicians. One source of the confusion is that the term stroke has been used in

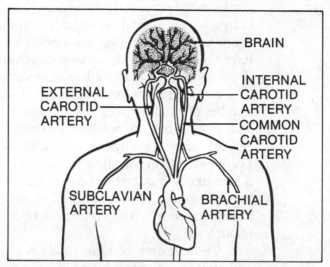

This illustration depicts the arteries that supply the brain with blood.

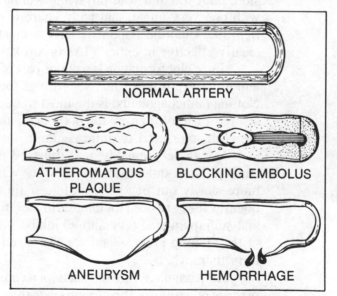

NORMAL ARTERY

ATHEROMATOUS PLAQUE

BLOCKING EMBOLUS

ANEURYSM

HEMORRHAGE

Strokes can be caused by atherosclerosis, which narrows the arteries and causes clots to form. If a clot blocks the blood flow to the brain, death of some of the brain tissue is the result.

Strokes can also result when a weak point in a cerebral blood vessel forms a bulge (aneurysm) and then bursts.

several different ways. It is more common for strokes to be preceded by transient ischemic attacks (TIAs)—neurological problems (such as weakness in one arm) that come and go—and/or for a patient to have several smaller stroke episodes over a period of days or weeks. This has led some physicians to refer to a series of TIAs as an "impending stroke" and to a number of small strokes as a "stroke in progress." But TIAs often do not lead to stroke, and most strokes occur as single events without additional symptoms before or after. In learning about TIAs and stroke, it may be helpful to remember that all of these situations represent a lack of adequate blood flow to the brain. The concern is to do something about that.

The question of *what to do* is controversial. Different treatments have been proposed for TIAs and strokes of various types. In making your decision, both you and your physician will have to deal with one very unpleasant fact: There has been no rigorous, scientific demonstration that any therapy is clearly effective in either TIAs or strokes.

Since clot formation is a major part of the problem in many strokes, the use of drugs that prevent clotting (anticoagulants) is the most frequently considered form of therapy for both TIAs and stroke. Heparin, one kind of anticoagulant, must be injected, acts very quickly, and must be monitored closely. Oral anticoagulants such as warfarin act more slowly but persist for a longer time. Consequently, they are used for long-term therapy. Aspirin and sulfinpyrazone (Persantine) inhibit one portion of the clotting process and are also used for long-term therapy.

Anticoagulants are not used for a cerebral hemorrhage or a ruptured aneurysm since they will make the bleeding worse. A special X-ray procedure called computerized tomography (CT or CAT scan) usually can distinguish between a stroke caused by clotting and one caused by hemorrhage. This procedure has become routine before starting anticoagulant drugs for a stroke.

Surgery may be performed in an effort to prevent stroke. This kind of surgery is difficult at best, and often simply impossible. However, there are several instances when surgery is undertaken:

- It is sometimes done when a bleeding aneurysm is relatively easy to reach.
- Microsurgery to relieve a blocked vessel inside the skull has been experimented with, but it is not an accepted therapy except in very rare cases.
- Surgery can be done much more easily on the large arteries (carotid arteries) in the neck that supply blood to the brain.

Surgery to remove a blockage in a carotid artery (endarterectomy) is the most common surgery done to prevent stroke, but such blockages are not common causes of stroke. Thus, surgery offers little to most threatened by stroke.

Deciding who has an obstruction of the carotid and might benefit from endarterectomy is not easy. Such obstructions may cause sounds called *bruits* that can be heard with a stethoscope placed over the carotid. But a bruit does not indicate the amount of obstruction; indeed, bruits may occur with no obstruction at all. In the past, arteriography (a special X-ray procedure requiring injections into the carotid) was the only way to determine the amount and location of blockage. However, this procedure carried a substantial risk of stroke and death. Fortunately, new techniques of determining blockages do not require injection into the carotid and do not carry these risks.

Benefits

Research on treatment for TIAs and stroke is difficult for a variety of reasons, some of which are discussed above. As a result, we have no scientific proof that any treatment is of substantial benefit. However, there *are* studies that provide information as to probable effects of treatment.

Findings from several studies suggest that the use of aspirin in a patient with TIAs will decrease the risk of subsequent stroke. Other studies have suggested that the same may be true for sulfinpyrazone (Persantine) and warfarin.

Most physicians believe that anticoagulation with heparin should be used if the symptoms of a stroke appear to worsen and a CT scan shows no evidence of hemorrhage in the brain. Heparin is also often recommended when the cause of the stroke is a clot that formed in the heart and was transported by blood flow to the brain (cerebral embolization). Because of the risk of cerebral hemorrhage, some physicians confronted with this situation will wait for 48 hours after embolization to administer heparin. Again, the available studies weakly support the use of anticoagulation drugs in these situations even though they do not conclusively demonstrate that patients will benefit.

Carotid endarterectomy is of unknown value in TIAs and is almost never performed during or after a stroke (see page 172). However, many physicians believe that patients will have fewer TIAs after an endarterectomy is performed if there is a high degree of blockage in the carotid artery (greater than 80 percent) *and* the symptoms can be attributed to the problem in the carotid. Remember that many people have blockage of the artery but either have no symptoms or their symptoms are related to another problem. Finally, if the blockage shows signs of breaking down (this is referred to as "ulcerated plaque" or ulceration), many physicians believe that this poses the same risk as a high degree of blockage.

There is no evidence that a carotid endarterectomy benefits patients who have no TIAs or other symptoms but who do have some evidence (e.g., bruit, etc.) of obstruction in the carotid.

Risks

The risks of aspirin therapy are related to its potential for causing allergic reactions (e.g., asthma-like attacks) or for irritating the stomach. The dose recommended for TIAs is quite low, so that irritation problems are unusual; allergy to aspirin is also infrequent. The possibility of excessive bleeding on this low-dose therapy is so small that it does not raise the risks of aspirin therapy significantly. Likewise, the risks (e.g., allergic reactions) of sulfinpyrazone are very small.

The main risks of heparin and warfarin therapy are excessive bleeding, which may present as cerebral hemorrhage; bleeding from the gastrointestinal tract; or blood in the urine. The risk of trauma due to injuries (auto accident, etc.) is also increased because of the possibility of massive bleeding. Five percent to 10 percent of patients taking heparin or warfarin will have minor bleeding episodes (nosebleeds, etc.), while approximately 0.5 percent to 1 percent will have major bleeding episodes. The risk of death due to bleeding is probably less than one in 1,000.

The risk of death during a carotid endarterectomy ranges from as low as 1 percent in major medical centers to as high as 20 percent in some community hospitals. The risk of stroke during the procedure is approximately the same.

Costs

The average hospital stay for strokes of all levels of severity is ten days. This average includes patients who had complications as well as those who were "routinely" admitted to the hospital for several days.

The cost of hospitalization for a stroke will depend on the length of stay. It conceivably could be as low as $2,000; it could be $8,000 or higher. Of course, the cost of medical care varies considerably from one region of the country to another, and your final bill could be above or below this range.

No one wants to sit idly by while TIAs or strokes get worse. At the same time, the lack of clear-cut benefits makes it necessary to focus on the risks of various approaches.

The available information suggests that there is no benefit to treating those obstructions of the carotid artery that do not cause symptoms. If there are no symptoms, it is probably best to forget about it, although aspirin or sulfinpyrazone may be considered.

Initial investigations of TIAs should include examination of the carotid arteries with tests such as oculoplethysmography or computerized digital subtraction angiography that do not require injection into the carotid artery. If a high degree of obstruction or ulceration of the carotid artery is found *and* the symptoms can be reliably related to the problem in the carotid, then a carotid endarterectomy may be considered. The only situation that routinely meets these criteria is transient blindness in the eye that is on the same side as the problem in the carotid. Otherwise, if TIAs have just begun, they may be treated with warfarin; after two months, drug treatment may be switched to aspirin. If the TIAs began *more than* two months ago, the patient may be started immediately on aspirin. Neither the diagnostic tests nor anticoagulation therapy require hospitalization.

It is not unusual for patients who suffer minor strokes to wait until several days or weeks have gone by before consulting a physician. Hospitalization seems to offer little in this situation since both tests and therapy can be accomplished without admission.

If a stroke has just occurred, hospitalization will be required if there is significant disability. Theoretically, a patient seen immediately after a mild stroke might not be hospitalized since the CT scan and other tests, as well as medical therapy, may be done on an ambulatory basis. In practice, the patient is almost always admitted to make it easier to get the tests done and easier to monitor the heparin therapy and the condition of the patient. Physicians, patients, and patients' families are all uneasy about "doing nothing" in the face of a stroke. Hospitalization is doing something, but it may be a more effective treatment for anxiety than for a mild stroke.

Once in the hospital, getting out as soon as you are able is the most important thing for your health. Anticoagulation therapy, physical therapy, etc. can all be done at home. Remember the rule: The problems caused by a stroke will get better regardless of therapy, and the most important influence on recovery is the degree to which the patient can experience a normal life.

Stroke

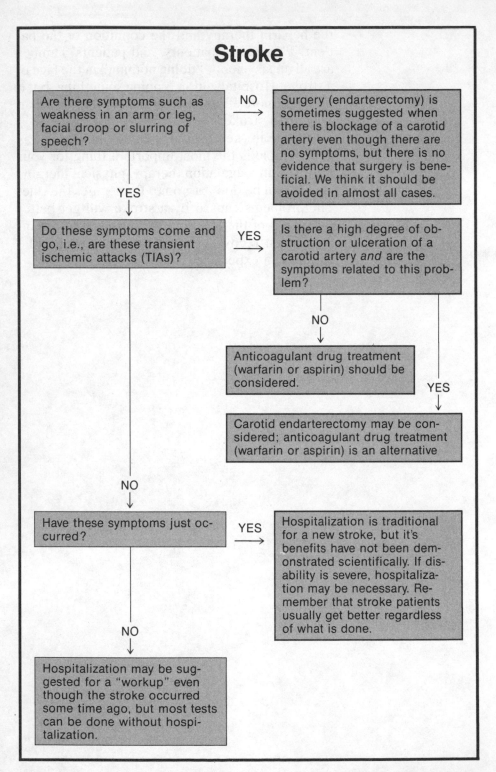

Are there symptoms such as weakness in an arm or leg, facial droop or slurring of speech?

→ NO → Surgery (endarterectomy) is sometimes suggested when there is blockage of a carotid artery even though there are no symptoms, but there is no evidence that surgery is beneficial. We think it should be avoided in almost all cases.

YES ↓

Do these symptoms come and go, i.e., are these transient ischemic attacks (TIAs)?

→ YES → Is there a high degree of obstruction or ulceration of a carotid artery *and* are the symptoms related to this problem?

NO ↓

Anticoagulant drug treatment (warfarin or aspirin) should be considered.

YES ↓

Carotid endarterectomy may be considered; anticoagulant drug treatment (warfarin or aspirin) is an alternative

NO ↓

Have these symptoms just occurred?

→ YES → Hospitalization is traditional for a new stroke, but it's benefits have not been demonstrated scientifically. If disability is severe, hospitalization may be necessary. Remember that stroke patients usually get better regardless of what is done.

NO ↓

Hospitalization may be suggested for a "workup" even though the stroke occurred some time ago, but most tests can be done without hospitalization.

24

Infections

Before antibiotics were available, infections were the leading cause of admissions to the hospital. Treatment consisted of good nursing care, keeping wounds clean, draining abscesses when appropriate, and controlling fever if possible. These indirect methods of fighting infection were often unsuccessful, but there was no alternative.

The advent of antibiotics made it possible to attack directly the organisms that cause many infections. Infections such as pneumococcal pneumonia that once were frequent reasons for admission to the hospital (and often killed their victims) became rare reasons for admission. Today patients with infections generally are admitted for only two reasons: (1) Severe illness requires intensive care in addition to antibiotics or (2) the antibiotics necessary require parenteral administration. Parenteral administration usually refers to intravenous or intramuscular injection, but on occasion may indicate direct injection into other portions of the body such as direct placement of antibiotics into the cerebrospinal fluid (intrathecal injection). Parenteral administration is most often required when the infection is difficult to eradicate and poses a serious threat to the patient; the most common examples are infection of bone (osteomyelitis) and infection of the heart (endocarditis).

Advances in home health care now allow many patients requiring parenteral therapy to leave the hospital. These patients are stable and not seriously ill, but do require frequent or continuous intravenous or intramuscular therapy. In the past, they stayed in the hospital at great cost and some risk to themselves simply because this was the only place in which the nursing skills and equipment were available. Now many areas have home health care services which provide these services effectively and efficiently, allowing the patient to lead a much more normal life.

There are limits to the types of services that home health care can provide, of course. Specifically, the more unusual types of parenteral therapy may not be available in the home. This is an area of rapid technological advances, so it is worthwhile pursuing the question of home therapy any time the patient is stable and not seriously ill but requires continuing treatment.

Benefits

Faith in antibiotics as wonder drugs should not obscure the very real threats of certain types of infections. The hospital's accepted role is to provide intensive care in addition to antibiotic therapy when patients are seriously ill. Such intensive services are usually required for a relatively short period.

The hospital's benefit when the patient is stable but requires continuing therapy is less clear. As indicated above, home health care agencies can now duplicate many of the services previously available only in the hospital.

The many types of infections and the generally accepted use of the hospital for seriously ill patients makes scientific evaluation of the benefits of hospitalization difficult. There is little information that compares hospital treatment for seriously ill patients with infections to other alternatives. Studies that compare home health care to hospital care for patients who are stable but require continuing parenteral therapy have not been done frequently, but they suggest that home health care is at least as effective as hospital care.

Risks

For the seriously ill patient, the risks of hospitalization are those associated with the use of multiple medicines and the other inherent risks of hospitalization. The stable patient who continues to be hospitalized for long-term parenteral therapy is also subject to the inherent risks of hospitalization, especially those due to inactivity.

Costs

The average hospital stay for people with infections is seven days. This average includes people whose hospital stays were longer than optimal because of complications or because they were "routinely" admitted to the hospital for several days.

If you are hospitalized for an infection, you can expect your bill to be between $2,000 and $5,000. The longer you stay in the hospital, the higher it will be. The cost of medical care varies from one region of the country to another, and your final bill could be above or below this range.

Making Decisions About Infections and the Hospital

Use of the hospital for the seriously ill patient with an infection clearly makes sense. Once the crisis has passed, the goals of medical care must include minimizing the risks posed by hospitalization. Since home health care agencies now can provide most types of intravenous and intramuscular therapy, discharge from the hospital as soon as possible is a reasonable goal for patients who are stable and not seriously ill. Patients requiring other types of parenteral therapy or with special requirements may not be suitable for home care, but this is a rapidly changing area and new services are becoming available. A thorough discussion of the costs, risks and benefits of home care with your physician and the home care agency is a necessity. If the physician is unfamiliar or inexperienced with respect to home care, a second opinion will be useful.

Infections

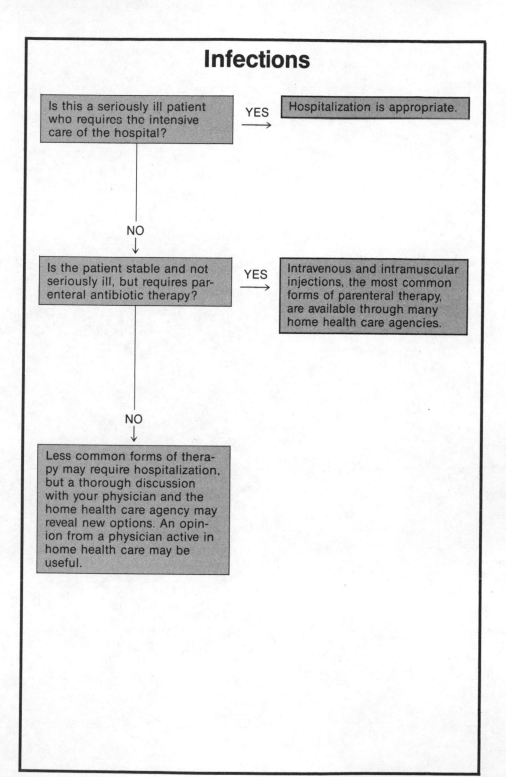

Is this a seriously ill patient who requires the intensive care of the hospital?

YES → Hospitalization is appropriate.

NO ↓

Is the patient stable and not seriously ill, but requires parenteral antibiotic therapy?

YES → Intravenous and intramuscular injections, the most common forms of parenteral therapy, are available through many home health care agencies.

NO ↓

Less common forms of therapy may require hospitalization, but a thorough discussion with your physician and the home health care agency may reveal new options. An opinion from a physician active in home health care may be useful.

Part VI

CHILDBIRTH

Good books on almost every aspect of childbirth abound, and expectant parents have months to read them. We have decided, therefore, to concentrate on the decisions parents face regarding hospitalization for childbirth and possible Caesarean delivery. Many parents are not aware that there are alternatives to the traditional hospital delivery. Often a mother does not know that the reason she has been given for needing a Caesarean section is not a valid one. The information provided here should help parents make appropriate choices and, it is hoped, help to decrease the number of unnecessary Caesarean sections that are performed.

25
Childbirth

Our attitudes toward childbirth have undergone two dramatic but gradual shifts since World War II. The forties and fifties saw increasing emphasis on use of the hospital for safe and painless childbirth. The key to improving the health of mothers and their babies was to bring the tools of modern medicine—drugs, machines, and surgery—to bear, using medical procedures to improve upon a natural event. Or so we thought.

The sixties and seventies saw the beginning of fundamental changes in these attitudes. We realized that safe and rewarding birth experiences depend more on the basic health of the mother and the prenatal care she receives than on the medical technology available at the time of the birth. Participation by mothers *and* fathers replaced "painless" as the goal for childbirth in the minds of many. To some, the hospital now seemed a hostile environment that did not provide warmth and support for this most intimate experience. As a result of this shift, births at home began to increase after declining for many years. The use of nurse midwives also increased in

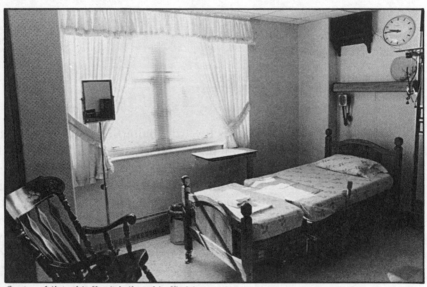

Courtesy of Alexandria Hospital, Alexandria, Virginia

A birthing room can help provide a warm, supportive environment for a very personal event.

popularity, and nurse midwives themselves have enjoyed increased professional acceptance.

Nevertheless, most babies are still delivered in hospitals by doctors. This undoubtedly reflects the desire of most Americans to use the best that modern medicine has to offer. But there have been significant changes. Most hospitals try very hard to make care of the mother and child less impersonal and to allow more participation by father and family. Many have developed birthing centers as units separate from the usual labor and delivery facilities of the hospital. The atmosphere of a birthing center is more like that of a hotel with nurses than that of a hospital. The rooms are more comfortable, family and friends may be with mother during labor and may be present at birth. Some birthing centers are designed so that labor and delivery occur in the same room while others use a more standard delivery room for the birth itself. The full range of hospital services is immediately available should they be needed. In most birthing centers, the care of the mother and child is under the direction of either a physician or a nurse midwife using a physician as a consultant.

Birthing centers may be located outside the hospital as well. Those located away from hospitals are more likely to emphasize the natural aspects of childbirth, and care is more likely to be under the direction of a nurse midwife. However, arrangements for immediate access to medical care are always made. Having the best of both worlds is central to the birthing center concept: a warm and supportive environment for an intensely personal event, but with the best of medical help available if needed.

Benefits

There is general agreement that the hospital offers substantial benefit when the delivery is complicated. The most obvious and frequent example is the need for delivery of the baby through an incision in the abdominal and uterine walls—a Caesarean section (usually referred to as a "C-section" in medical jargon). However, there has been increasing concern that many Caesarean operations are unnecessary. In the past, a large number were done simply because a previous delivery had been by this method. Physicians feared that a uterus weakened by a previous Caesarean birth might rupture during labor. It is now known that this is very unlikely and that a normal, vaginal delivery is appropriate if there are no other problems that prohibit it.

The vast majority of deliveries are natural and uncomplicated and do not require the services of the hospital. Moreover, most deliveries that *will* require the services of the hospital can be identified well in advance of birth during prenatal examinations by the physician. Thus, the key to using the hospital wisely is adequate prenatal care. The benefits of using a birthing center or delivering at home are determined largely by the value placed on these settings by the mother and father. For an event of this importance, these benefits may be considerable. Birthing centers and the home may also avoid the inherent risks of the hospital, especially in terms of infection.

Risks

The risk of the mother's death during childbirth is estimated to be less than one in 10,000. The risk of death to the baby just before or after birth is a little more than one in 100. *But* we do not have information on how the risk differs for deliveries done in homes versus birthing centers versus hospitals. Also, because complicated deliveries are much more likely to end up in the hospital than in a birthing center or at home, it is quite likely that hospitals have higher death rates simply because they have most of the patients who suffer complications. There is no scientific information that would allow us to separate out the inherent risks of hospitalization.

The risks of a birthing center or home delivery must also be considered. Assuming that prenatal care has been adequate and that a normal delivery is expected, the principal risk is that of an unexpected complication such as uncontrolled bleeding. Again, there have been no scientific studies that tell us what this risk is. We do know that these problems are more likely to occur, and that labor is more likely to be prolonged, with first pregnancies than with subsequent ones.

Costs

In the case of a normal delivery with no complications, the optimal hospital stay is one day. If birth occurs before noon, often mother and child can go home later that same day. In the case of a Caesarean birth with no complications, the optimal stay is three days. Currently, the average hospital stay for a normal delivery is three days. For a Caesarean, it is six days. These averages include women whose hospital stays were longer than optimal because of complications or because they were "routinely" admitted to the hospital for a specified number of days.

The average cost for a normal delivery is $2,054. Caesareans average $3,300. It should be kept in mind that medical care costs vary considerably between different regions of the country, and your final bill could be higher or lower.

Making the Decision About Childbirth and the Hospital

The two factors that can best help you choose an appropriate setting for childbirth are adequate prenatal care and understanding your own needs. If prenatal examinations indicate that a normal, vaginal delivery is expected, then delivery at a birthing center or at home are options. However, the mother will want to take certain precautions if she has had a previous Caesarean section.

The American College of Obstetricians and Gynecologists (ACOG) recently revised its guidelines for vaginal birth after Caesarean (VBAC) and reconfirmed the safety and advisability of vaginal birth for the vast majority of women.

ACOG recommends that hospitals offering VBAC be prepared to start emergency Caesarean surgery and anaesthesia within 30 minutes of the time the decision is made. The previous recommendation was for surgery to begin within 15 minutes. As precautionary measures, continuous fetal monitoring and 24-hour access to blood-bank facilities are advised.

VBAC is not recommended in every case. For example, women who have had more than one Caesarean birth or who are carrying more than one infant or a single infant estimated to weigh more than nine pounds are advised not to attempt it.

Currently, as many as one in five births are by Caesarean section in the United States. This figure is considerably higher in some hospitals. Twenty-five to 30 percent are performed because the mother has previously given birth by this method. Comparisons with other countries indicate that this figure is unnecessarily high. In England, a country with a lower infant mortality rate than the United States, only 12 percent of mothers who have had a Caesarean *will* have a Caesarean for subsequent delivery.

ACOG estimates that at least 80 percent of women who attempt trial labor will be successful if the recommended guidelines are followed. Interested prospective parents should discuss the procedure with their obstetrician. If a Caesarean is recommended simply because the mother has had one before, the parents should get a second opinion.

There is certainly nothing wrong with trying to have the best of both worlds. For this reason, birthing centers deserve your consideration. This option may be both more comfortable and less expensive than the hospital. We believe it should be no more risky than the other options, and we hope that it may be even less risky.

Finally, if you should choose a hospital or birthing center, stay only as long as you must in order to avoid the inherent risks of inactivity and infection. This does not mean that you should equate returning home with a return to the full range of activities that you were involved in before delivery. Indeed, support at home is the key to getting the care you need after childbirth without the risks of hospitalization. Help and support at home are important for dealing with the blues that often follow delivery as well.

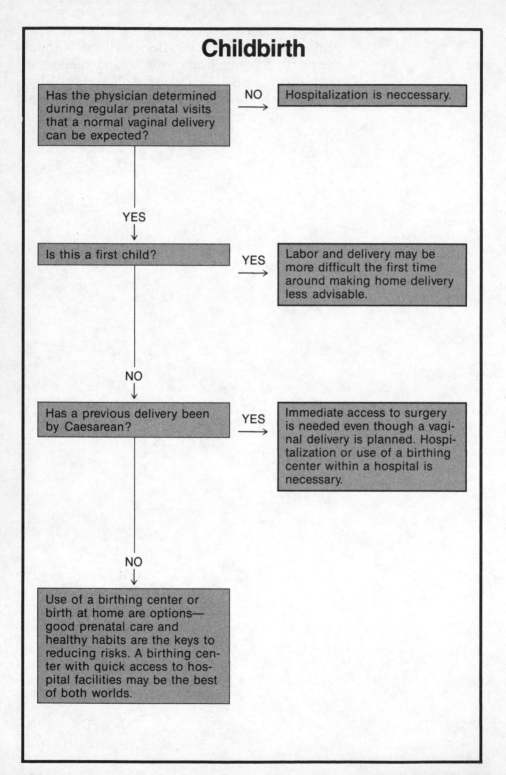

Childbirth

Has the physician determined during regular prenatal visits that a normal vaginal delivery can be expected?

NO → Hospitalization is neccessary.

YES ↓

Is this a first child?

YES → Labor and delivery may be more difficult the first time around making home delivery less advisable.

NO ↓

Has a previous delivery been by Caesarean?

YES → Immediate access to surgery is needed even though a vaginal delivery is planned. Hospitalization or use of a birthing center within a hospital is necessary.

NO ↓

Use of a birthing center or birth at home are options—good prenatal care and healthy habits are the keys to reducing risks. A birthing center with quick access to hospital facilities may be the best of both worlds.

Part VII

PSYCHIATRIC ADMISSIONS

Sometimes people are admitted to the hospital because they are determined to be in need of psychiatric help or because they are suffering a severe problem related to drug or alcohol abuse. In all of these cases, hospitals are equipped to provide short-term care by preventing disturbed people from harming themselves or others, by providing medical care and observation to people suffering from overdoses or withdrawal episodes, and by treating the severe complications of substance abuse.

The long-term supervision and therapy that all of these people require must be sought outside the hospital. However, a number of hospitals employ counselors to help patients make contact with sources of long-term treatment.

26
Psychosis and Depression

Psychosis is a general term for mental disorders in which the patient's thinking seems irrational and detached from reality. In the past, the lack of effective treatment for such problems made it necessary to concentrate on limiting the harm of irrational behavior. In many cases, this meant placement in a chronic-care institution (asylum). In other cases, the patient remained at home to be cared for and supervised by family and friends. The hospital played little role in the care of such patients, occasionally holding patients until they could be transferred elsewhere.

The advent of effective antipsychotic drugs changed the situation dramatically. Although the exact actions of these drugs on the brain is still unknown, it is clear that they are able to reduce or eliminate psychotic behavior in many patients. These drugs gave the hospital a new role in the care of these patients: They could provide short-term care until drugs could relieve psychotic symptoms, and the patient could be transferred to an ongoing program of care outside the hospital. Today many hospitals have psychiatric wards specifically organized for this purpose.

Not all psychotic patients require hospitalization. In deciding on hospitalization, the key determination is whether or not the patient presents an immediate threat to himself or herself or to others. It is not unusual for a psychotic individual to function well at home, at work, and in the community. It is important to distinguish between behavior that is unusual or makes others uncomfortable and that which presents a danger.

Depression is the other major reason for use of the psychiatric facilities of the hospital. Again it is the question of danger—in this case the risk of suicide—that determines whether or not the hospital is well used. Antidepressant drugs may be helpful in severe depression, but their effectiveness is less predictable than that of the antipsychotic drugs. It is also true that the immediate threat of suicide may lessen rather rapidly with nondrug therapy, or simply with the passage of time if the patient can be prevented from harming himself or herself at the critical point.

Patients who do not present danger to themselves or others usually do not benefit from the short-term care available in the hospital. If continuing supervision or intensive therapy is deemed appropriate for such patients, it is best to look for these services outside of a hospital. Day-care programs in which the patient is treated and supervised during the day but returns home at night are often useful and have become increasingly popular. A residential program at a special facility may also be worthwhile, but this tends to be expensive and may not prepare the patient to re-enter life outside the residential facility.

Decisions with respect to the risk of doing harm or the need for supervision are often difficult. Using the hospital or the residential facility when unsure about the need for supervision is understandable, of course. At the same time, it is important to remember that the long-term care of these patients is likely to be outside the hospital or residential facility. Most important, it must be recognized that there is no way in which these decisions can be made perfectly.

Indeed, it is often difficult to determine whether choosing one alternative over another made any difference in how the patient fared in the long run.

Benefits

There is little information available on the effectiveness of hospitalization in preventing harm to patients or to others. There are depressing statistics suggesting that unsuccessful suicide attempts are likely to be followed by successful ones. This does not give information on the hospital's ability to prevent suicide attempts in the first place or to prevent assaults on others. It does mean that neither hospital care nor other forms of medical care "cure" depression. Nevertheless, our society believes that the hospital represents the most intensive care available and that this level of care is appropriate when a life is at stake. In view of this, it seems unlikely that we will soon see studies that compare hospital treatment to other alternatives for the care of patients who are judged to be dangerous or suicidal.

Controversy continues as to whether residential programs or day programs provide benefits beyond those of drugs. Unfortunately, there is not sufficient scientific data to allow a determination of the benefit of such programs.

Costs

The average hospital stay for problems of psychosis and depression is 15 days. This average includes hospital stays that were longer than optimal because of complications or delay in finding more appropriate methods of treatment.

The cost of hospitalization for psychosis or depression will probably range between $2,000 and $13,000. The size of the bill is largely determined by the length of stay. However, the cost of medical care varies from one region of the country to another, and your final bill could be above or below this range.

Making Decisions About Psychosis or Depression and the Hospital

The hospital is the place for short-term care that is aimed at preventing harm to the patient or to others. It is not the place for long-term care, nor is it appropriate for psychiatric problems that do not require intensive monitoring.

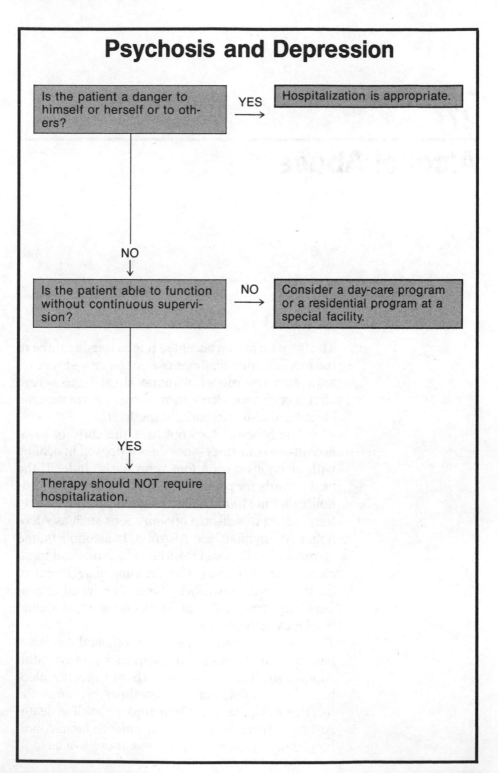

Psychosis and Depression

Is the patient a danger to himself or herself or to others?

YES → Hospitalization is appropriate.

NO ↓

Is the patient able to function without continuous supervision?

NO → Consider a day-care program or a residential program at a special facility.

YES ↓

Therapy should NOT require hospitalization.

27
Alcohol Abuse

The hospital has an accepted role in treating three of the medical complications of alcoholism—severe intoxication (overdose), withdrawal, and the severe effects of chronic alcoholism such as gastrointestinal bleeding due to cirrhosis of the liver.

The hospital does not have the cure for alcoholism—no one does—nor does it do well in dealing with alcoholism on a long-term basis. Indeed, the best records for producing lasting results with alcoholism are not found within the medical community; they belong to self-help organizations such as Alcoholics Anonymous and Al-Anon. In alcoholism, the hospital is really a last resort in which medical treatment is used to deal with an immediate threat of death or severe disability. It is not designed to provide long-term treatment for alcoholism and should not be expected to do so.

Getting drunk, sleeping it off, and having a hangover have been experienced by most adult Americans. The frequency with which acute alcoholic intoxication occurs sometimes obscures the fact that it is quite possible to drink yourself to death. Although there is no specific antidote for alcohol, life-support procedures, such as those available in most intensive care units, can be essential in such a situation.

While the familiarity of terms such as sleeping it off and hangovers suggests that recovery from alcohol intoxication is routine, many of us are aware also that severe withdrawal symptoms may occur when the steady, excessive use of alcohol is stopped abruptly. Convulsions and the spectacular delirium tremens (DTs)—a semi-comatose state with continual shaking of the body that may last for days—are some of the complications that may occur during withdrawal. While there are no treatments that will absolutely prevent withdrawal or its complications, there are medicines that can reduce its severity. General life-support measures are also important in weathering the crisis of withdrawal.

Some hospitals have organized their services for acute alcoholism into units called alcohol detoxification ("detox") units. Such units recognize that acute alcoholic problems are common and that the services required for their treatment are somewhat different from those usually provided in either intensive care units or a standard hospital ward. Many detox units also emphasize counseling with the objective of connecting the alcoholic patient with a source of long-term treatment. This recognizes that the successful resolution of an overdose or withdrawal episode does not do anything for the basic problem of alcoholism and that dealing with alcoholism requires a long-term approach outside the hospital.

Some hospitals have gone one step further than the detoxification unit and provide up to several weeks of behavioral and psychiatric therapy aimed at dealing with the basic problem of alcoholism. These services are usually referred to as alcohol treatment units (ATUs); they are controversial, primarily because they are expensive and cannot provide long-term care. Their supporters argue that the ATU is valuable in beginning the process of successful treatment and that this treatment can then be carried on outside the hospital. Others believe that the ATU is useful for a patient who is unstable and may be a threat to himself or herself or to others, but that it offers little advantage in other circumstances.

Cirrhosis and damage to the nervous system are the most severe effects of chronic alcoholism. Coma and gastrointestinal bleeding are devastating complications of cirrhosis that must be treated in a hospital. The tragic truth is that treatment of these complications may prevent an immediate death, but does nothing to resolve the underlying problems. It often seems that long and very expensive hospitalizations do little more than save the patient so that he or she may drink again with the inevitable result of more complications and eventual death.

Benefits

No scientific studies compare the hospital treatment of alcohol overdose or withdrawal to out-of-hospital treatments, simply because no one is willing to treat such serious problems outside the hospital. Nevertheless, there is general agreement among physicians that the use of the hospital's specialized services is effective and can prevent death or serious complications.

Similarly, there is little disagreement over the treatment of the severe complications of chronic alcoholism such as gastrointestinal bleeding or coma. Common sense seems to dictate that the chances of successful treatment are best in the hospital despite the lack of scientific studies to confirm this.

The use of expensive hospital facilities for counseling and psychiatric therapy aimed at changing alcohol behavior is less clear. No studies have demonstrated that prolonged hospitalization has any advantage over other approaches, provided that the patient can be maintained in the home and community and does not need the medical treatment that can only be found in the hospital. Indeed, as indicated before, the best records for long-term treatment of alcoholism lie with self-help groups. The use of an ATU for patients who are unstable and may be threats to themselves or others seems rational but has not been studied scientifically.

Risks

The lack of studies concerning hospitalization for acute alcohol problems does not allow the specific probabilities of complications to be assigned to these admissions. The risks are those associated with hospitalization and the use of drugs, primarily the drugs used in treating the complications of withdrawal.

The risks of hospitalization for the complications of chronic alcoholism are even more difficult to determine because the risks of death are so great regardless of what is done. For example, one study of gastrointestinal bleeding found that medical (supportive) therapy was associated with a mortality rate of 11 percent while surgical therapy was associated with a mortality rate of 18 percent. Surgery is usually done only if medical therapy fails. Neither approach will cure or prevent recurrence. Finally, it is important to note that it has been estimated that only 10 percent of persons with severe cirrhosis will survive for five years.

Costs

The average hospital stay for problems of alcohol abuse is 11 days. This average includes hospital stays that were longer than optimal because of complications or delay in finding more appropriate methods of treatment.

The cost of hospitalization for alcohol abuse will probably range between $2,000 and $9,000. The size of the bill is determined primarily by the length of stay. However, the cost of medical care varies from one region of the country to another, and the final bill could be above or below this average.

Making Decisions About Alcohol Abuse and the Hospital

Despite the lack of scientific studies, it seems clear that the person with a potentially lethal overdose of alcohol or someone who is in danger of going into withdrawal should be treated in the hospital. If a detoxification unit is available, all the better.

Likewise, the treatment of the severe complications of chronic alcoholism demands hospitalization simply because the chances of survival outside the hospital seem so low.

The use of the hospital for the primary treatment of alcoholic behavior is expensive and seems less effective than the alternatives when the patient can live at home and function in the community. The ATU may play a role for patients who are a risk to themselves or others. A residential program in a special facility may be reasonable if the patient is unlikely to do harm but is unable to live at home.

Alcohol Abuse

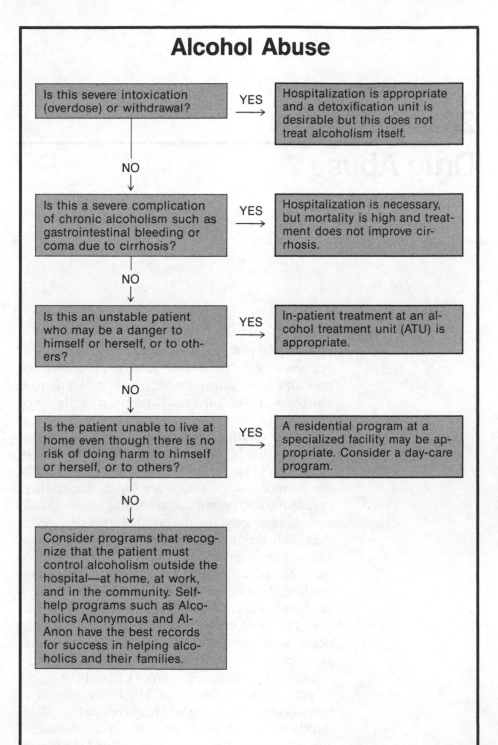

Is this severe intoxication (overdose) or withdrawal?

YES → Hospitalization is appropriate and a detoxification unit is desirable but this does not treat alcoholism itself.

NO ↓

Is this a severe complication of chronic alcoholism such as gastrointestinal bleeding or coma due to cirrhosis?

YES → Hospitalization is necessary, but mortality is high and treatment does not improve cirrhosis.

NO ↓

Is this an unstable patient who may be a danger to himself or herself, or to others?

YES → In-patient treatment at an alcohol treatment unit (ATU) is appropriate.

NO ↓

Is the patient unable to live at home even though there is no risk of doing harm to himself or herself, or to others?

YES → A residential program at a specialized facility may be appropriate. Consider a day-care program.

NO ↓

Consider programs that recognize that the patient must control alcoholism outside the hospital—at home, at work, and in the community. Self-help programs such as Alcoholics Anonymous and Al-Anon have the best records for success in helping alcoholics and their families.

28
Drug Abuse

The hospital plays a more limited role in dealing with the abuse of drugs such as sedatives (barbiturates, methaqualone, diazepam, etc.) and opioids (heroin, morphine, methadone, etc.) than it does in the abuse of alcohol. Its major role is preventing death from an overdose or during withdrawal. Occasionally, it may be used to hold an unstable patient who may be dangerous to himself or herself or to others. Finally, the hospital may be necessary for the treatment of certain medical complications of drug abuse, usually serious infections. But the hospital is not designed to deal with the underlying problem of drug abuse. Indeed, the availability of drugs in the hospital and the potential for manipulation of hospital personnel by the drug abuser make the hospital a particularly poor environment in which to deal with drug abuse.

The most dangerous drug overdoses usually occur with sedatives and opioids, but they may also occur with stimulants (amphetamines, etc.), cocaine, and hallucinogens (LSD, PCP, etc.). There are medicines that block the effects of opioids and others that will help reduce the effects in other types of overdoses. However, the use of any of these medicines is complex, and the patient may require life-support measures as well. These usually necessitate intensive care in the hospital.

Withdrawal from barbiturates is an extremely serious problem and carries the risks of convulsions and death. Withdrawal from opioids produces a myriad of physical and psychological symptoms, but convulsions and death are not seen in this situation. Withdrawal from stimulants produces relatively mild physical symptoms, but psychological problems may be profound. Stopping the use of cocaine, hallucinogens, and marijuana may produce psychological and emotional problems, but they do not produce the life-threatening physical problems seen in withdrawal from barbiturates or alcohol.

Successful treatment of an overdose or withdrawal does nothing for the underlying problems of drug abuse. Occasionally, a patient may be treated successfully for drug overdose or withdrawal, but remain a threat to himself or herself or to others. In such a situation, the hospital may provide a safe place where the patient can stay while treatment for these problems is begun and transfer to an appropriate program can be accomplished.

Few topics are more controversial or have received more attention in the media than the treatment of drug abuse. Given the many types of drug abuse and the many types of individuals involved in it, it is safe to say that no one program will be demonstrated to be effective for this widespread problem. It is also safe to say that effective programs must have a long-term approach and that the hospital is simply not the place for this type of treatment.

Benefits

Because our current understanding of overdose and withdrawal seems to demand treatment in the hospital, scientific studies have not compared the hospital treatment of these problems to alternatives. While it is well known that withdrawal from opioid or stimulant addiction may be accomplished without medical supervision, this alternative is unlikely to be tested in a scientific manner because of ethical and legal considerations. The hospital appears to be necessary to save some individuals from death due to overdose or during withdrawal; the vast majority of physicians are unwilling to attempt any other mode of treatment.

Using the hospital as a safe place to hold a patient who appears to be a danger to himself or herself or to others is justified by the same concerns; there is no scientific study available that compares hospital to nonhospital treatment.

Even the most widely recognized long-term programs for drug abuse lack complete scientific evidence of their effectiveness. The hospital seems particularly unlikely to be successful in this area since it is not organized for long-term care of complex psychosocial problems. Given this, it is not surprising that there is no evidence of the hospital's effectiveness in dealing with this problem.

Risks

Without specific scientific studies on the use of the hospital for drug abuse, it must be assumed that the risks of hospitalization are those associated with the intensive care facilities. These may carry a risk of death as high as 1 percent or more, but this is difficult to evaluate against a background of the very high risk posed by the overdose or withdrawal situations themselves.

Costs

The average hospital stay for problems of drug abuse is 12 days. This average includes hospital stays that were longer than optimal because of complications or delay in finding more appropriate methods of treatment.

The cost of hospitalization for drug abuse will probably range between $2,000 and $10,000. The size of the bill is determined primarily by the length of stay. However, the cost of medical care varies from one region of the country to another, and the final bill could be above or below this range.

Making Decisions About Drug Abuse and the Hospital

It seems clear that the hospital is the place for patients who are suffering from a drug overdose or withdrawal, or who present a danger to themselves or others. At the same time, the hospital is not the place for dealing with the basic problem of drug abuse. The most useful thing that the hospital can do once the immediate danger has passed is to guide the patient into a recognized and respected continuing treatment program outside the hospital.

Table 28.1 Symptoms and Signs of Drug Abuse

HALLUCINOGENS
(LSD, psilocybin, mescaline, PCP, STP, MDMA, Bromo-DMA)

Signs of Severe Intoxication	Symptoms of Withdrawal
Pupils dilated	None
Rapid pulse	
Elevated blood pressure	
Face flushed	
Visual hallucinations	
Distorted vision and sense of time	
Slurred speech	

With PCP:
Extreme hyperactivity
Drooling
Impulsive, often violent behavior

CENTRAL NERVOUS SYSTEM STIMULANTS
(Amphetamines, cocaine, methylphenidate, phenmetrazine, phenylpropanolamine, most anti-obesity drugs)

Signs of Severe Intoxication	Symptoms of Withdrawal
Pupils dilated	Muscle aches
Rapid pulse	Abdominal pain
Shallow breathing	Chills and tremors
Hyperactive, easily excitable behavior	Intense hunger
Rapid speech	Extreme depression
Dry mouth	Anxiety
Sweating	Increased sleep
Impulsive behavior	Suicidal behavior

CANNABIS SUBSTANCES
(Marijuana, hashish, THC, hash oil)

Signs of Severe Intoxication	Symptoms of Withdrawal
Bloodshot eyes	Irritability
Increased appetite	Anxiety
Euphoria or anxiety	Nausea
Dreamy, fantasy state	Inability to sleep
Time-space distortions	Restlessness
Increased heart rate	

OPIOIDS-NARCOTICS

(Heroin, morphine, codeine, meperidine, methadone, hydromorphone, opium, pentazocine, propoxyphene)

Signs of Severe Intoxication

Pupils constricted
Reduced breathing rate
Decreased body temperature
Reflexes diminished or absent
Decreased blood pressure

In overdoses:
Stupor or coma
Convulsions

Symptoms of Withdrawal

Abdominal cramps
Muscle jerks
Flu symptoms
Vomiting
Diarrhea
Trembling
Anxiety

CENTRAL NERVOUS SYSTEM SEDATIVES

(Barbiturates, chlordiazepoxide, diazepam, flurazepam, glutethimide, meprobamate, methaqualone)

Signs of Severe Intoxication

Decreased blood pressure
Reduced breathing rate
Slow motor reflexes
Drowsiness or coma
Loss of muscular coordination
Slurred speech
Delirium

Symptoms of Withdrawal

Trembling
Sweating
Collapse of cardiovascular
  system
Delirium
Hallucinations
Disorientation
Inability to sleep

ANTICHOLINERGICS

(Atropine, belladonna, henbane, scopolamine, trihexyphenidyl, benztropine mesylate, procyclidine, propantheline bromide)

Signs of Severe Intoxication

Pupils dilated and fixed
Increased heart rate
Temperature elevated
Flushed, dry skin and mucous
  membranes
Confusion
Visual hallucinations

Symptoms of Withdrawal

Gastrointestinal disorders
Musculoskeletal disorders

Adapted from *The Medical Letter on Drugs and Therapeutics,* Vol. 27 (Issue 696), September 1985. Published by The Medical Letter, Inc., New Rochelle, New York.

Drug Abuse

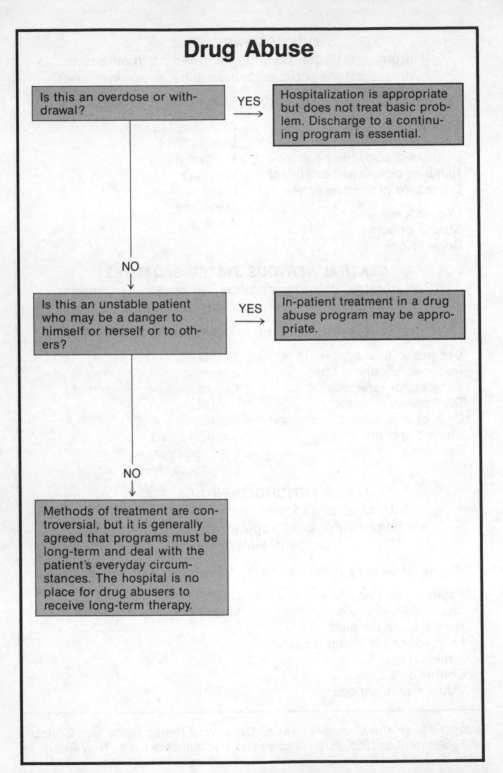

Is this an overdose or withdrawal?

YES →

Hospitalization is appropriate but does not treat basic problem. Discharge to a continuing program is essential.

NO ↓

Is this an unstable patient who may be a danger to himself or herself or to others?

YES →

In-patient treatment in a drug abuse program may be appropriate.

NO ↓

Methods of treatment are controversial, but it is generally agreed that programs must be long-term and deal with the patient's everyday circumstances. The hospital is no place for drug abusers to receive long-term therapy.

Part VIII

SUMMING UP

The procedures and treatments described in this book are just some of the invaluable services that modern hospitals provide. But it is essential that hospitals be used appropriately, and this requires informed patients.

If you have read Parts I, II, and III of this book, great! You have prepared yourself to be an informed patient. If the question of hospitalization comes up, you have some understanding on which to base your decisions, and you know where to turn:

- To the chapters in this book that deal with specific problems
- To doctors
- To friends and family
- To organizations that provide information and support.

The Taking Part Check List that follows should help you make certain you have covered all the important questions pertaining to hospitalization.

Now, if you are faced with a decision about using the hospital, have confidence in yourself and remember the "Golden Rule": Avoid the hospital when you can, know what's happening when you can't.

The Taking Part Check List

Use these questions as a guide to decision making about the hospital.

Yes	No	
____	____	Are the tests, procedures, or therapy necessary?
____	____	Can they be performed outside the hospital?
____	____	Have the benefits, costs, and risks of hospitalization been explained?
____	____	Do you understand your right to accept or reject health care on the basis of your own personal values and in furtherance of your own personal goals (informed consent)?
____	____	Is testing recommended simply because it is routine? (This is not an acceptable indication for testing.)
____	____	Are drugs used only when needed?
____	____	Has a second opinion been obtained?
____	____	Have the benefits, costs, and risks of surgery been explained?
____	____	Can the surgery be done on an ambulatory basis?
____	____	Are you seeking to use the hospital for an inappropriate reason, as for a rest?

Glossary

A

Adenoidectomy	Surgery to remove the adenoids.
Adhesions	Fibrous scar bands that join together body tissues that are normally separate.
Ambulatory	Surgery or a procedure that does not require a stay in the hospital; walk-in or outpatient surgery.
Anaesthesia	Total or partial loss of sensation, usually artificially induced.
Anaesthesia, General	Total loss of sensation, i.e., unconsciousness, usually produced by inhaling an anaesthetic gas.
Anaesthesia, Local	Regional loss of sensation, i.e., only in the operative site.
Anaesthesiologist	A physician who administers anaesthetics.
Aneurysm	A weak point in a blood vessel that forms a bulge. When that bulge bursts, it is called a ruptured aneurysm.
Angina Pectoris	Severe constricting pain in the chest, usually caused by coronary disease.
Antibiotics	Drugs used to treat infections by destroying or inhibiting the growth of microbes.

Anticoagulants	Substances that prevent clotting.
Antihistamines	Drugs that reduce the symptoms of colds or allergies counteracting the effects of histamine, a chemical involved in allergic reactions.
Appendectomy	Removal of the appendix (organ of the lower gastrointestinal tract).
Arteriography	Visualization of an artery by X-ray after injection of a contrast agent.
Arthroscope	An instrument used to examine the insides of joints.
Arthroscopy	Examination of the inside of a joint.

B

Biopsy	The process of removing tissue from living patients for diagnostic testing.
Bruit	Abnormal sounds within an internal organ or body part, usually arising from turbulent blood flow in an artery.

C

Caesarean Section	Delivery of a baby through an incision in the abdominal and uterine walls.
Carotid Arteries	Large arteries in the neck that supply blood to the brain.
Carotid Endarterectomy	The surgical excision of the inner lining of a clogged carotid artery.
Cartilage	Semi-rigid connective tissue; some types of cartilage act as a shock absorber between bones.
Cataract	A cloudiness that forms in the lens of the eye.
Cataract, Congenital	A cataract present at birth.
Cataract, Traumatic	A cataract that occurs as a result of injury.
Cerebral Embolus	A blood clot that has been transported by blood flow to the brain.
Cerebral Hemorrhage	Bleeding into the brain.

Cerebral Infarction	Death of brain tissue caused by blockage of blood flow to the brain.
Chemotherapy	The treatment of disease with chemicals.
Cholangiograms	X-ray of the bile ducts after injection with a contrast medium ("dye").
Cholecystectomy	Surgical removal of the gallbladder.
Cholecystitis	Inflammation of the gallbladder.
Cholecystotomy	An incision into the gallbladder to allow drainage.
Chronic Diseases	Prolonged, lingering diseases, such as diabetes and arthritis.
Cirrhosis	A chronic disease of the liver marked by progressive destruction and degeneration of liver cells that ultimately results in death.
Common Duct	The tube that collects the secretions of the pancreas, liver, and gallbladder and delivers them to the intestine.
Computerized Tomography (CT Scan)	A complex X-ray procedure in which an image of a cross-sectional plane of the body is generated by computer synthesis.
Congenital	Existing at birth.
Contrast Agents	Chemical substances that are injected or ingested during the X-ray procedure in order to make certain body structures visible on the X-ray.
Coronary Artery Bypass Grafting (CABG)	Surgery on the coronary arteries, which supply blood to the heart—a vein from another part of the body (usually the leg) is used to bypass a blocked portion of the coronary artery. By attaching that vein above and below the obstruction, blockages caused by coronary artery disease can be bypassed.
Coronary Artery Disease	Disease of the arteries supplying the heart.
Coronary Care Unit	A special section in the hospital reserved for patients who require care for heart disease.
Coronary Occlusion	Blockage of a coronary blood vessel that can lead to heart attack.

Cryoextraction	The use of a freezing probe to remove lens of the eye in a cataract operation.
Cystic Duct	The tube leading from the gallbladder to the common duct that allows bile to leave the gallbladder.
Cystocele	Hernia of the bladder.

D

Dehydration	Loss of body fluids.
Diabetes	A chronic disease characterized by inadequate production of insulin or resistance to insulin.
Diagnosis	The act or process of identifying or determining the nature of a disease through history and examination.
Disc, Herniated; Disc, Slipped	When a vertebral disc bulges out and presses on the nerves as they leave the spinal cord.
Discs, Vertebral	Discs of cartilage that separate the bones in the back.

E

Electrocardiogram	A graphing of the heart's electric currents.
Embolism	Obstruction of a blood vessel by a detached clot, air bubble, or other foreign body.
Endocarditis	Inflammation of the endocardium, the membrane that lines the heart.
Eustachian Tube	The passage that leads from the ear to the throat.
Extracapsular	Outside of the capsule or covering membrane.

F

Fluoroscope	A fluorescent screen on which the internal organs may be continuously viewed by transmission of X-rays through the body.
Fluoroscopy	Examination with the use of a fluoroscope.
Foot Drop	Paralysis or weakness of the muscle function of the leg and foot, which causes the foot to fall and the toes to drag on the ground when walking.
Fusion Procedure	Permanently joining bones together.

G

Gallbladder   An organ located in the upper gastrointestinal area that stores bile, a mixture of substances produced by the liver that aids in the digestion of food.

Gallstones   Crystals in the gallbladder, created when the liver secretes an abnormal bile that contains too much cholesterol relative to the other chemicals present (e.g., bile salts and phospholipids).

Gallstones, Silent   Gallstones that cause no symptoms in the patient (usually found via X-rays, surgery, or post mortem).

Gastrointestinal (GI)   Relating to the stomach and intestines.

Graft   Any unattached tissue or organ that can be used for transplantation; also the actual transplantation.

H

Hematocrit   The percentage of blood that is composed of red blood cells.

Hernia   A protrusion or bulging of a body tissue through the structure that contains it.

Hernia, Femoral   A bulging in the groin area, lower than an inguinal hernia.

Hernia, Incarcerated   A condition in which an organ is trapped in the hernia sac and unable to return to the abdomen.

Hernia, Inguinal   A bulging through a weak portion of the abdominal wall in the groin area.

Hernia, Strangulated   A condition in which an organ is trapped in the hernia sac in such a way that the blood supply to the organ is shut off.

Hernia, Umbilical   A bulging around the umbilicus, or belly button, usually seen in children.

Holter Monitor   A small device that can make, on magnetic tape, a continuous recording of the heartbeat (electrocardiogram) for 24 hours or more. The patient can wear the monitor as he or she goes about normal activities at home or work.

Hypnotics — Medications causing sleep.

Hysterectomy — Surgical removal of the uterus.

I

Indications — Appropriate reasons for use of a treatment.

Informed Consent — When a patient, conscious and clear of mind, gives the provider of care his or her approval for the care to be given.

Intensive Care Unit — A specialty unit of the hospital for care of seriously ill patients containing special medical equipment and services.

Internist — A physician who specializes in the treatment of nonsurgical diseases in adults.

Intracapsular — Within a capsule or covering membrane.

Intramuscular (IM) — Within a muscle (e.g., IM injection).

Intraocular — Within the eyeball.

Intrathecal — Within the sheath covering the spinal cord.

Intravenous (IV) — Within a vein or veins.

L

Laparotomy — Surgical incision into the abdominal wall.

Ligaments — Tough, fibrous bands of tissue connecting bones or cartilage or supporting an organ or muscle.

Lumpectomy — Surgical removal of a tumor, in addition to some surrounding tissue, from the breast; local resection.

Lymphoid — Tissue that pertains to the lymphatic system, makes antibodies and plays an important role in developing immunity.

M

Mastectomy — Surgical removal of the breast.

Mastectomy, Radical — Surgical removal of the breast, pectoral muscles, and surrounding lymph nodes.

Mastectomy, Simple	Surgical removal of the breast tissue only.
Mastectomy, Total	Surgery in which all breast tissue and adjacent lymph nodes are removed, but the muscles of the chest (pectoral muscles) are not disturbed.
Myelogram	Visualization of the spinal cord by X-ray after the injection of a contrast agent.
Myocardial Infarction	Death of heart muscle; a heart attack.
Myringotomy	A small hole placed in the eardrum to allow fluid to drain; a small tube is sometimes placed in the hole to keep the passage open.

O

Oculoplethysmog-raphy	Measuring and recording changes in the pressure within the eyes; a method of testing circulation to the eye and brain.
Oncologist	A medical doctor specializing in tumors.
Osteomyelitis	Inflammation of the bone marrow and surrounding tissues.

P

Palate	The roof of the mouth.
Pancreas	A long, soft, irregularly shaped gland lying behind the stomach; secretes pancreatic juice, a secretion containing enzymes that aid in digestion, and produces insulin.
Pancreatitis	Inflammation of the pancreas.
Parenteral	The introduction of substances into the body in a manner other than by mouth (i.e., intravenous, subcutaneous, intramuscular, etc.)
Pathology	The medical science that deals with all aspects of disease.

Percutaneous Transluminal Coronary Angioplasty (PTCA)	A procedure designed to relieve blockage in the coronary artery. A balloon tipped catheter is passed into a large artery, usually in the groin, and then maneuvered to the site of narrowing of the coronary artery. By inflating the balloon, the artery is dilated and the blockage is relieved.
Phacoemulsification	The use of ultrasound to liquify the lens (used in cataract operations).
Postoperative Care	The care a patient receives following an operation.
Preoperative Care	The care a patient receives prior to an operation.
PRN	An abbreviation for the Latin *pro re nata,* meaning according to need. These initials used in orders for medication mean that medication is given only if the patient requests it or the nurse believes it necessary.
Procidentia	A sinking down or prolapse of the uterus.
Prognosis	A forecast of the probable outcome of a disease.
Prosthesis	An artificial device used to replace a breast, limb, or other body part.
Puerperal Sepsis	Childbed fever.
Pulmonary Embolus	A blood clot carried by the circulating blood to the lungs.

R

Rectocele	Prolapse or herniation of the rectum.
Rheumatology	The study of various conditions related to the joints and muscles.

S

Sciatica	Pain, numbness, and/or weakness radiating down the leg to the foot caused by pressure on the sciatic nerve.
Sprain	An injury to a joint with partial tearing of a ligament or tendon.

Stroke
Sudden occurrence of unconsciousness, paralysis, weakness or other symptoms resulting from a cerebral hemorrhage or the blocking of a blood vessel that supplies the brain.

Surgicenters
Centers that are separate from a hospital and that are designed, staffed, and organized specifically for the purpose of performing ambulatory surgery.

T

Thrombophlebitis
Inflammation within the veins, usually accompanied by clot formation.

Tonsillectomy
Surgery to remove the tonsils.

Truss
A pad attached to a belt and held in place by straps or a spring that is used to prevent the return or enlargement of a hernia.

V

Vital Signs
The temperature, pulse, respiratory rate, and blood pressure of an individual.

Index

general, *See* General anaesthesia
for hernia operation, local vs. general,
73–74
local, *See* Local anaesthesia
risks, 126
types, 61
Anaesthesiologist, 50, 60
Anal fistulectomy, 31t
Anemia, from gastrointestinal bleeding,
151
Aneurysm
bleeding, surgery for, 167
ruptured, stroke from, 164, 165, 166
Angina, angina pectoris, 139
coronary artery bypass grafting for,
104–105, 108
distinguished from myocardial
infarction, 141
hospitalization for, for testing, 142
symptoms, 140
Angiogram, 30t
Antibiotics, 14, 173
parenteral administration, 173–174,
175, 177
Anticholinergics, intoxication and
withdrawal, 207t
Anticoagulants, 166
heparin, 166, 168, 169
warfarin, 166, 168, 169
Antidepressant drugs, 192
Antihistamines, 58
Anti-obesity drugs, abuse, 206t
Antipsychotic drugs, 191
Appendicitis, 149
hospitalization for, length of stay, 150
Arteries, *See also* specific artery
hardening of, *See* Atherosclerosis
Arteriography, 167
coronary, 107
Arthritis, 159
Arthrogram, 30t
Arthroscopy, 30t
knee, 123, 124, 125, 126
costs, 126
Arthrotomy, 126
Aspirin therapy, for TIA and stroke,
risks, 166, 168–169
Asylum, *See* Chronic-care institution
Atherosclerosis, stroke from, 164, 165
Atropine, 207t
Attending physician, 48
Attitudes, patient, 7
ATUs, *See* Alcohol treatment units

B

Baby, death, 184
Back surgery, 96
benefits, 98
costs, 99
decision-making, 99–101
reasons for, 96, 98
risks, 99
Bacteria, 14
Barbiturates, 58, 202
intoxication and withdrawal, 203t
symptoms and signs, 207t
reactions to, 16
Bed rest, 15, *See also* Inactivity
hazards, 142
for low back pain, 155, 156
Behavioral therapy, for alcoholism,
197–199
Belladonna, 207t
Benefits of hospitalization, 7, 8, *See
also* under specific heading
Benztropine mesylate, 207t
Bile, 87, 88
Biopsy, 30t
for breast cancer, 118, 122
Birthing center, 183, 184, 186, 188
risks, 184–185
Birthing room, 182
Bladder control, loss of, 158
Bleeding, *See also* Hemorrhage
active, emergency room care for, 42
from anticoagulant therapy, 169
gastrointestinal, *See* Gastrointestinal
bleeding
rectal, 151
Blepharoplasty, 30t
Blood, vomiting of, 151, 152
Blood clot
formation, and stroke, 165, 166
heart, 168
leg, 125
Blood pressure, 56
Blood tests, 53, 55, 141
Breast cancer, 116
biopsy for, 118, 122
mastectomy for, *See* Mastectomy
prognosis, 119
Breast tissue, removal, *See* Mastectomy
Breath, shortness of, emergency
room care for, 43
Bromo-DMA, 206t
Bronchoscopy, 30t
Bruit, 167

Bunionectomy, 30t

C

CABG, *See* Coronary artery bypass
    grafting
CAD, *See* Coronary artery disease
Caesarean section, 179, 183
   costs, 185
   length of hospital stay, 185
   necessity, 183–184
   rates, 186
   vaginal birth after Caesarean (VBAC),
     185–186
Cancer
   breast, *See* Breast cancer
   gallbladder, 89
   ovaries, 132, 133–134
   uterus, 132
Cannabis substances, intoxication and
    withdrawal, 206t
Cardiac catheterization, 30t
Cardiologist, 65
Carotid arteries
   blockage, 167, 168
   surgery, 167
Carotid endarterectomy, 168, *See also*
    Endarterectomy
   risks, 169
Carpal tunnel release, 30t
Cartilage, knee
   removal, 126
   surgery, decision-making, 127, 128
   tears, 125
Case, knowledge of, 19
CAT, *See* Computerized tomography
Cataracts, 109
   extraction (surgery), 30t
     advances, 109, 111
     on ambulatory basis, 113, 115
     benefits, 112
     contact lenses following, 111
     costs, 113
     decision-making, 113–115
     intraocular lens following, 111
     length of hospital stay, 113
     procedure, 111
     results, 111–112
     risks, 112–115, 116
     types, 112
     vision following, 113, 115
Catheterization, cardiac, 30t
CCU, *See* Coronary care unit
Central nervous system

sedatives, *See* Sedatives
stimulants, *See* Stimulants
Cerebral embolization, 168
Cerebral hemorrhage, stroke from, 164,
   166
Cerebral infarction, 164
Check list, survivor's, 209, 211
Chemotherapy
   combined with lumpectomy, 118
   combined with mastectomy, 119
Chenodeoxycholic acid, 89
Chest
   muscle, removal, 120
   pain, 139, 140, *See also* Angina;
     Myocardial infarction
    hospitalization for costs, 144
    decision-making, 144–145, 146
   X-rays, 55
Chief resident, 49
Childbed fever (puerperal sepsis), 13
Childbirth, 179, 180, *See also* Caesarean
    section
   attitudes toward, 181
   birthing center, 183, 184, 186, 188
    risks, 184–185
   birthing room, 182
   at home, 181, 184, 188
    risks, 184–185
   home support following, 187
   hospitalization for, 183
    benefits, 183–184
    costs, 185
    decision-making, 185–188
    length of stay, 185
    for prenatal care, 184, 185
    risks, 184
Children, hernias in, 75–76
   inguinal, 79, 80
   umbilical, 80, 81
Chlordiazepoxide, 207t
Cholangiogram, 90
Cholecystectomy, 90, 91, 92
   costs, 92
   risks, 92
Cholecystitis
   acute, 90
   chronic, 90
   diagnosis, 94
   hospitalization for
    length of stay, 150
   recurrent, 91
   surgery for
    benefits, 91
    decision-making, 92–93, 95

risks, 92
Cholecystostomy, 90–91
Choosing of hospital, 66–67
Chronic care institution (asylum), for
   psychosis, 191
Chronic diseases
   goal of treatment, 159
   hospitalization for, 159
      benefits, 161
      choosing of hospital, 66
      decision-making, 162–163
      reasons, 159–161
      risks, 161–162
Circulatory system
   healthy, 15
   injection through, *See* Intravenous
Cirrhosis, from alcoholism, 198
   hospitalization for, 201
   period of survival, 199
Clots, *See* Blood clots
Cocaine, 202
   intoxication and withdrawal, 203
      symptoms and signs, 206t
Codeine, 207t
   reactions to, 16
Cold sweat, emergency room care for,
   43
Collateral ligaments, tear, surgery for,
   125
   decision-making, 126–128
Colonoscopy, 30t
Common duct exploration, 91
Community hospital, 48, 66
Computerized tomography (CT, CAT),
   and stroke, 166
Congestive heart failure, 159
Consent, 7, 19
   informed, 20–22
Constipation, 60
Consultants, 51
Contact lenses, following cataract
   surgery, 111, 115
Contrast agents, allergic reactions to, 17
Coronary artery(ies), 103
   blockage, 139, 140
Coronary artery bypass grafting
   (CABG), 102, 103f, 105
   costs, 106
   decision-making, 107
   length of hospital stay, 106
   reasons for undergoing, 104–105
Coronary artery disease (CAD), 102
Coronary care unit (CCU), 8, 141
   benefits, 142–143

length of stay, 141, 142, 146
   risks, 143
   transfer from, 144
Costs, *See also* under specific heading
   emergency room, 41–42
   of hospitalization, 7, 8–9
Counseling, for alcoholism, 198
Cruciate ligaments, surgery on, 123
Cryoextraction of cataract, 109, 111, 112
C-section, *See* Caesarean section
CT, *See* Computerized tomography
Cystic duct, 91
Cystoscopy, 30t

D

Dalmane, 58
Day-care programs, for psychosis and
   depression, 192, 193, 195
D&C, *See* Dilatation and curettage
Death, *See also* Death rate; Sudden
   death newborn, 184
Death rate
   associated with hospitalization, 8
   for chronic disease, 162
   from back operations, 99
   from cholecystectomy, 92
   decrease in, 8
   from hernia operation, 78
   from heart surgery, 106
   from tonsillectomy and
      adenoidectomy, 84
Decision, decision-making, *See also*
   under specific heading
   for ambulatory surgery, 40
   analysis, 77
   doctor, 50
   for emergency room care, 42–43
   for hospitalization, 2, 211
      survivor's rules for, 11–12
   patient's competence in, 22
   shared, 21–22, 50, 51
Decision maker, patient as, 6
Dehydration, 149, 152
   hospitalization for, 150–151
Demands, unreasonable, 23
Depression, *See also* Suicide
   antidepressant drugs for, 192
   day-care program for, 192, 193, 195
   hospitalization for, 192, 193
      benefits, 193
      costs, 193
      decision-making, 194–195
      length of stay, 193

residential programs for, 193, 195
Dermatologist, 65
Detecatest, 151
Diabetes, 159
  hospitalization for, 160
Diagnosis, hospitalization for, 4
Diagnostic tests, *See also* Laboratory
    tests; Blood tests
  outpatient, 4, 5
Diarrhea, 152
Diazepam (Valium), 58, 202, 207t
Diet(s), 63
Dietician, 53–54
Dilatation and curettage (D&C), 30t, 132
Disc
  herniated, 71, 98
  material, removal of, 98
  slipped, 98
  surgical removal, 99
  space, narrowing of, 155
  vertebral, 96, 97
Discharge from hospital, timing for, 10
Disease, *See* Chronic diseases
Disorientation, emergency room care
    for, 43
Diuretics, thiazide, reactions to, 16
Doctor(s), *See also* Medical staff
  attending physician, 48
  choosing of, 64–66, 67
  family, 147
  on hospital staff, 47
    interns and residents, 48–49
  "personal," 49
  primary care, 64
  as resource, 24–25
  rounds, 57
  specialists, 65, 67
  types of practices, 65
  working with, 50–51
Doctor's orders, 20
Drowsiness, emergency room care for,
    42
Drug(s), *See also* specific drug
  abuse, *See* Drug abuse
  antibiotics, *See* Antibiotics
  anticoagulant, *See* Anticoagulants
  antidepressant, 192
  for gallstones, 89
  intravenous and intramuscular
      injection, 60
  laxatives, 60
  overdoses, 202, *See also* Drug abuse
    hospitalization for, 208
    treatment, 203

for pain, 59–60
  reactions to, 8, 16
  risks, 16–17
    reduction of, 19
  sleeping pills, 57
  withdrawal, 203
    treatment, 203
Drug abuse
  hospitalization for, 202–203
    benefits, 203–204
    costs, 204–205
    decision-making, 205, 208
    length of stay, 204
    risks, 204
  long-term therapy, 208
  symptoms and signs, 206–207t
Dyes, allergic reactions to, 17

E

Ear infection, adenoidectomy for, 86
Eardrum, surgery, *See* Myringotomy
Ectopic pregnancy, 149
Elastic stockings, 16
Electrocardiogram, 2, 139, 141
Embolism, emboli, pulmonary, 15, 16,
    125
Embolization, cerebral, 168
Emergency patient, admission, 9
Emergency room, 27, 41–42
  care, 7
    decision-making, 42–43
Emphysema, 159
  hospitalization for, 160
Endarterectomy, 167
  carotid, 168
  risks, 169
ENT specialist, 65
Esophageal spasm, 142
Esophagogastroduodenoscopy, 31t
Exercise, 15
Extracapsular cataract surgery, 113
Eye surgery, *See* Cataract

F

F.A.C.S., 66
False negative readings, 18
False positive readings, 18
Family, as resource, 24, 25–26
Family physician, 147
Fellowship, 67
Femoral hernia, 73
  operation for, 80

Pancreatitis, 94
Parenteral administration, *See also*
    Intramuscular injection;
    Intravenous, injection
  of antibiotics, 173–174, 175, 177
Pathologist, 50
Pathology, 45–50
Patient
  attitudes, 7
  emergency, *See* Emergency patient
    responsibilities, 6–7, 20, 22–23
  rights
    informed consent, 20–22
    principle, 22
  role, 6
  view on hospitalization, 6
PCP, 202, 206t
Pediatrics, 67, *See also* Children
Penicillins, reaction to, 16
Pentazocine, 207t
Percutaneous transluminal coronary
    angioplasty (PTCA), 104
  decision-making, 107, 108
  risks, 105–106
Persantine, *See* Sulfinpyrazone
Personnel, *See* Hospital staff
Phacoemulsification, 30t, 109, 112
Phenmetrazine, 206t
Phenylpropanolamine, 206t
Physical medicine, 50
Physician, *See* Doctor
Pilonidal cyst excision, 31t
Placebo effect, of heart surgery, 105
Plaque, ulcerated, 168
Pneumonia, pneumococcal, 173
Postoperative care, responsibility for, 10
Pregnancy, *See also* Childbirth
  ectopic, 149
Prenatal care, 184, 185
Primary care physician, 64
Private service, 48, 49
PRN order, 58–59
Procyclidine, 207t
Proctosigmoidoscopy, 31t
Propantheline bromide, 207t
Propoxyphene, 207t
Psilocybin, 206t
Psychiatric admissions, 189
  alcohol abuse, 196–201
  drug abuse, 202–208
  psychosis and depression, 191–195
Psychiatric therapy, for alcohol abuse,
    197–198
Psychosis, 191

antipsychotic drugs for, 191
  day-care programs for, 192, 195
  hospitalization for, 193
    costs, 193
    decision-making, 192, 194–195
    length of stay, 193
PTCA, *See* Percutaneous transluminal
    coronary angioplasty
Puerperal sepsis (childbed fever), 13
Pulmonary embolism, emboli, 15, 16
  from knee surgery, 125
  sudden death from, 15
Pulse, 56

Q

Questions, 11–12, 19, 51

R

Radiation, *See also* X-rays
  exposure, 17
  therapy
    combined with lumpectomy, 118
    combined with mastectomy, 121,
      122
Radiologist, 50
Rectum, passage of blood through,
    hospitalization for, 151
Resident(s), 48–49, 51
  chief, 49
Residential program
  for alcoholism, 200, 201
  for depression, 193, 195
Resources, 24
  doctors, 24–25
  family and friends, 25–26
  organizations, 26
Respiratory rate, 56
Responsibility
  assigning of, 22
  medical staff, 6–7
  patient, 7, 20, 22–23
  physician, 50
  for postoperative care, 10
Rest, 15, *See also* Bed rest; Inactivity
    hospitalization for, 12, 137, 161,
      163
Results, knowledge of, 69
Rhinoplasty, 31t
Risks, *See also* specific heading
  of hospitalization, 7–8, 10, 112, 142,
    156
  drugs, 16–17

Teaching hospital, 48, 49, 51, 67
Teaching service, 48, 49
Technicians, 53
Temperature, body, 56
Tenotomy, 31t
Tests, testing, *See also* Diagnostic tests
  acceptable indications, 211
  blood, 53, 55, 141
  hospitalization for, 137
  laboratory, *See* Laboratory tests
  risk, reduction of, 19
  survivor's rule, 55
  timing of, 56
THC, 206t
Therapy
  medical, *See* Medical therapy
  surgical, *See* Surgical admissions;
      Surgery
Thiazide diuretics, reactions to, 16
Thoracic surgeon, 65
Throat, sore, 84, 86
Thrombophlebitis, 15, 16
TIAs, *See* Transient ischemic attacks
Tonsil(s), 81, 82
  enlarged, 83
  function, 83
  size, 83
  surgery, *See* Tonsillectomy and
      adenoidectomy
Tonsillectomy and adenoidectomy
      (T&A), 30t, 31t, 81–82, 129
  benefits, 83–84
  costs, 84–85
  decision-making, 85–86
  risks, 84
Traction, for low back pain, 153, 154
Transient ischemic attacks (TIAs)
  hospitalization for, decision-making,
      170, 172
  initial investigation, 170
  stroke following, 166, *See also* Stroke
  treatment, 166, 168
    research on, 167–168
    risks, 168–169
Treatment options, 69
Trihexyphenidyl, 207t
Truss, for hernia, 74
Tubes, 61
"Tune-up," hospitalization for, 161, 163

U

Ulcer(s), length of hospital stay, 150
Ulcerated plaque, 158
Umbilical hernia, 71, 73, 80

  operation, 76
Uncertainty, 12, 22
"Uncertainty principle," and
    hospitalization, 6
Unconsciousness, emergency room care
    for, 42
Upper gastrointestinal tract, bleeding
    from, 149, *See also*
    Gastrointestinal bleeding
Urinalysis, 55
Urinary tract, infection, following
    hysterectomy, 133
Ultrasound, 110
Uterus
  anatomic relationship, 130
  cancer, 132
  removal, 131–132 *See also*
    Hysterectomy

V

Vaginal birth after caesarean (VBAC),
    185–186
Valium, *See* Diazepam
Varicocelectomy, 31t
Varicotomy, 31t
VBAC, *See* Vaginal birth after
    caesarean
Vertebrae, 97
Vertebral discs, 96, 97
Vision, following cataract surgery,
    111–112, 113, 115
Vital signs, checking of, 56–57
Volunteer organizations, as resource, 24
Vomiting, 150, 152, *See also* Nausea
  blood, 151, 152

W

Warfarin, and stroke, 166, 168
  risks, 169
Women, gallstones in, 89

X

X-ray(s), 49, *See also* Radiation
  chest, 55
  coronary arteriography, 107
  gallbladder, 90
  for low back pain, 155, 158
  risks, 17
    reduction of, 19
X-ray technician, 53

Y

Young people, shortness of breath, 43